KETO DIET

Cookbook for Women Over 50

Feel Young Like Never Before and Restart Loving You.
3 Weeks Meal Plan To Accelerate Weight Loss,
Delay Aging And Boost Your Metabolism | 300+ Recipe

BY
ADELE GLENN

Table of Contents

CHAPTER 13: DINNER RECIPES 84

CHAPTER 14: SOUP AND STEW 100

INTRODUCTION

Although most women gain weight when they get older, this isn't always the case. Step up your exercise level and eat a nutritious diet to avoid weight gain beyond 50. You may realize that maintaining your normal weight gets more challenging as you grow older. Many females gain weight when they approach menopause. However, weight growth beyond the age of 50 is not unavoidable. You may reverse the trend by focusing on good eating habits such as the Keto Diet and maintaining an active lifestyle.

What causes weight gain in women over 50 years?

In most cases, the weight increase is caused by age and lifestyle and hereditary factors. Muscle mass, for example, declines as people become older, but fat levels rise. The pace at which your body burns calories slows down as you lose muscle mass (metabolism). It may be more difficult to maintain a healthy weight due to this. You'll gain weight if you keep eating the same way you always do and don't improve your physical activity. Genetic factors might also influence weight growth. You're more prone to gain weight around the abdomen if your parents or other close relatives do. Other factors that lead to weight increase beyond a certain age include lack of exercise, bad food, and insufficient sleep. People who don't get enough sleep are more likely to snack and eat more calories. Weight gain later in life might have major health consequences. Excess weight, particularly around the middle, raises your risk of a variety of problems, including:

- Cardiovascular and vascular disease
- Breathing difficulties
- Diabetes type 2

Excess weight raises your chance of developing malignancies such as breast, colon, and endometrial cancers.

How to prevent weight gain after 50

There is no secret method for avoiding or reversing weight gain after menopause. Simply follow these weight-loss guidelines:

- **Eat less**

You may require around 200 fewer calories per day in your 50s than you needed in your 30s and 40s to maintain your present weight, much alone removing extra pounds.

- **Seek support**

Surround yourself with people who encourage you to eat well and exercise. Better yet, make the improvements together.

Remember that weight reduction takes lifelong adjustments in food and activity habits. Commit to a better lifestyle.

- **Move more**

Physical activity, such as aerobic activity and strength exercises, may aid in weight loss and maintenance. Your body will burn calories more effectively as you grow muscle, making it simpler to maintain a healthy weight. Experts suggest moderate aerobic exercise, such as brisk walking, for at least 2 hours per week for most healthy individuals, or strong aerobic activity, such as running, for at least 75 minutes per week for most healthy adults. Strength training activities should also be done at least twice per week. You may need to exercise more to shed weight or reach certain fitness objectives.

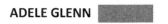

- **Check your sweet habit.**

Sugars add almost 300 calories to the typical American diet. Soft drinks, juices, energy drinks, flavored waters, and sweetened coffee and tea account for over half of these calories. Cookies, pastries, cakes, doughnuts, ice cream, and candies are also high in sugar.

- **Limit alcohol**

Alcoholic drinks are high in calories and increase the risk of weight gain.

Why is it so hard for women over 50 to lose weight?

Why are you gaining weight when you haven't altered your diet or workout regimen? A few often requested questions and tips for middle-aged ladies. Age-related loss of lean muscle mass lowers metabolism. We also tend to become less active, resulting in weight gain. Yes, even from fit patients. Women tend to notice the progressive weight increase around 40-50. They used to be able to skip a snack and lose weight. But now, the scale doesn't budge. Men lose muscle, and their metabolism decreases as they age. Women's hormones don't affect guys. Without estrogen, menopause causes a fat belly shift. Cardiovascular disease, strokes, and type 2 diabetes are increased by abdominal obesity.

Assuming you are similarly active, you require 200 fewer calories per day at 50 than you did at 20. Your caloric needs decrease beyond 60. Up to age 50, 2,000 calories per day is appropriate for moderate activity. After 50, stick to 1800 calories. Harder workers believe they are burning more calories than they are.

Contrary to common opinion, exercise alone will not significantly reduce weight. Also, working out times as hard might make you hungry and overeat. So experts don't advise double the workout to eat twice as much. Along with calorie reduction, 30-60 minutes of moderate exercise every day is advised.

How can you boost your metabolism?

Breakfast

It provides all-day energy. Breakfast deprivation increases hunger. Eating a big breakfast, a moderate lunch, and a light evening is ideal.

Strength-Training

It used to be purely cardio. Your metabolism is boosted as you gain muscular mass. Muscle mass decreases with age.

Lean Protein

Eat more lean protein, including fish, poultry, eggs, and tofu. You'll be fuller for longer, and your metabolism will be faster.

Are there specific foods you should never eat?

No such thing exists. You shouldn't feel deprived. Obviously, highly processed foods, fried foods, and alcohol should be avoided. Have it in modest doses. Processed foods like white flour and sugar induce blood sugar changes and hunger cravings. If you eat clean six days a week, take a day off. The following day, return to healthful eating.

Are there specific foods that can boost metabolism?

Spicy foods, including capsaicin from chili peppers, have been shown to increase metabolism. Hydrate well. Green tea may also aid metabolism.

What are some helpful tools?

Experts recommend Weight Watchers because it emphasizes portion management. Also, the My Fitness Pal app offers a free meal diary. It keeps you responsible and aware of what you consume. Fitbit's that monitor your exercise also assist.

- Heredity affects everything. A quick metabolism is partly hereditary. People who stare sideways at a doughnut gain weight. Some individuals will lose weight faster than others. What you have is all you have. It's hard not to feel disheartened when you're working so hard to lose weight. Maintain a healthy lifestyle and exercise consistently to lose weight.
- Sleep is vital to our weight. Sleep-deprived persons eat more calories and are more likely to be overweight. Sleep deprivation promotes hormonal imbalance and food cravings. We should all get up early.
- Antidepressants, steroids, diabetic drugs, and seizure medications are among the medications that might induce weight gain. They may cause fluid retention, slow metabolism, and increased hunger. If you keep gaining weight despite eating healthy and exercising, ask your doctor about your medications. Don't stop taking them, but ask your doctor if they're causing you to gain weight.

Your body adapts as you age, so does your nutrition. Aren't you what you eat? Eating healthy meals becomes even more critical for women over 50. Decades of study have equipped doctors with dietary information that may help women age gracefully. Experts advise women over 50 to priorities three key nutrients to fight normal aging changes.

Protein for healthy muscle mass

Women in their later years tend to sit more and exercise less. This accelerates the normal aging process of sarcopenia or the loss of muscular mass. By the time they reach the age of 80, women may have lost up to half of their skeletal muscle mass. Protein consumption helps to mitigate the effects of muscle atrophy. If you make smart choices, a healthy plant-based diet that excludes meat, a key source of protein, may nevertheless offer sufficient protein. More soy, quinoa, eggs, dairy, almonds, seeds, and beans are among the foods he advocates. Your protein requirements are determined by your weight. Experts suggest 1 to 1.5 grams of protein per kilogram of body weight (1 kilogram = 2.2 pounds) for women over 50. For example, if you weigh 140 pounds, you'll need at least 63 grams of protein every day.

Calcium for bone health

Osteoporosis is a serious bone condition that affects elderly women. Women over 50 are at risk of osteoporosis-related bone fractures. Men get osteoporosis, too, although not as often. Women consume less calcium as they grow older, and some women's ability to handle dairy, which is one of the finest sources of calcium, declines as well. Other acceptable options are dark leafy greens and calcium-fortified orange juice. Women over the age of 50 need 1,200 mg of calcium every day. Keep track of your consumption by reading the Nutrition Facts label on food goods.

Vitamin B-12 for brain function

Women absorb fewer nutrients from their diet as they age, according to experts. Vitamin B-12, which is necessary for both healthy blood cells and brain activity, is one important nutrient they may not be getting enough of. Eggs, milk, lean meats, fish, and fortified cereals and grains are the finest sources of vitamin B-12.

Vegans will need to pick fortified foods in particular, but even senior individuals who consume a varied diet may struggle to absorb enough vitamin B-12. While 2.4 mcg of vitamin B-12 per day is the recommended daily requirement for women over 50, experts recommend speaking with your doctor to determine whether you additionally need a supplement.

Three pieces of advice from experts to help women over 50 receive the nutrients they need.

- Make whole foods your diet's base. A diet rich in whole grains, fruits, and vegetables can help you prevent many of the difficulties that come with becoming older.

- Make a mealtime appointment. (And don't throw it away.) Experts often advise their patients to make precise strategies outlining how they will get vital nutrients. Make a calendar with the plan. You're more likely to eat that apple if you make an 'appointment' with it.

- Don't wait till you're thirsty to drink. As you become older, the way your body detects thirst changes. Even if you don't feel thirsty, be sure to drink lots of water. Carry a bottle of water with you and drink a glass of water with each meal.

Why Keto Diet is a Solution

The ketogenic diet requires you to make significant dietary modifications. Carbohydrates, such as bread, grains, cereals, and many fruits and vegetables, are severely restricted in this high-fat, low-protein diet. The keto diet might be difficult to stick to, but some individuals find that the advantages outweigh the difficulties when they do. The keto diet may be beneficial to those over 50 since it has the ability to improve weight reduction, blood sugar management and maybe protect against heart disease. However, there are hazards to this eating plan, and you must always see your doctor or a qualified nutritionist before beginning any new diet.

How Does the Keto Diet Work?

It's just a half-fast. When you consume carbohydrates, your blood sugar rises, and this sugar fuels the body's cells. When you don't consume carbohydrates for a long time, your blood sugar levels drop, and your liver starts to use stored body fat as a source of energy. It's similar to having a backup system for your body. Ketosis is the name for this process. Because the keto diet isn't a complete fast, your body still has a source of energy, and you may keep your muscle mass.

Foods You Can Eat on the Keto Diet

The keto diet consists of a high-fat, moderate-protein, and low-carbohydrate diet. Your body will reach a state of ketosis if you do this properly and regularly for 2-3 weeks. The keto diet follows a macronutrient ratio (fat, carbs and protein). Typical fat-to-protein-to-carbohydrate ratios are 4:1 or 3:1, which means your diet will have 4 or 3 g of fat for every 1 g of protein and carbohydrate combined. This equates to around 70% to 80% fat, 20% to 30% protein, and 10% to 15% carbohydrate. This equates to around 165 g of fat, 75 g of protein, and 40 g of carbohydrate in a normal 2000-calorie diet.

The foods you can eat on a keto diet include:

- Nuts
- Small amounts of meat and fish
- Cheese
- Seeds
- Dairy products
- Veggies
- Greek yogurt
- Eggs

Foods to Avoid on the Keto Diet

High-carbohydrate foods are forbidden from the diet. Here are a few examples:

- Fruits. (Because of their great nutritional content, berries may be tolerated in little doses.)
- Legumes and beans
- Refined and unrefined grains, as well as starches (such as cereals, bread, pasta, wheat, rice, rye, potatoes, barley, starchy vegetables)
- Foods that have been processed

Benefits of the Keto Diet

Weight reduction is one of the first things that many individuals will notice on a diet. However, a large portion of it is due to water weight. Sugar is linked with water and stored in your body. As a result, when you eliminate carbohydrates, your body consumes the sugar and releases the water, giving the illusion of weight reduction. Other advantages of the keto diet, other than weight loss, include:

Heart health is important: The keto diet may lower total cholesterol and raise "good" (HDL) cholesterol levels in certain people. This might help reduce your chances of developing heart disease.

Controlling blood sugar levels: Lower blood sugar levels have been related to diet.

Keeping your lean body mass: It's typical to lose muscle mass and feel weaker as we get older. Because you'd be receiving more protein and restricting bad foods on the keto diet, you could be able to preserve muscle for longer.

Is the Keto Diet Safe After 50?

It might be if you do so under the supervision of your doctor, so check with them first. If your doctor prescribes you the go-ahead, make sure you're getting enough rest and drinking enough water to be hydrated. Inquire with your doctor about how to maintain a healthy balance of essential nutrients while being on the keto diet. Taking vitamin and fiber supplements may be necessary. Losing and weight maintenance beyond 50 is difficult, but if you stay motivated and stick to the Keto diet, you will succeed.

CHAPTER 1:

WHAT IS THE KETO DIET?

Keto diets are a diet that produces ketones at its heart. Ketones are formed when so few carbohydrates exist that energy must be extracted when fatty acids are broken down. A few different diets, including the adapted Atkins diet, the Atkins diet, and the ketogenic diet, fall within this broad umbrella of low carb diets.

You eat very high fat and low carbohydrates in the mainstream, conventional ketogenic diet. The rest is protein. The ratios are roughly 75% fat, 20% protein and just 5% carbohydrates.

The Atkins diet allows only carbohydrates to be counted, which makes maintenance easier. "You're getting 20 or fewer grams, and that's it. The fat and protein count is not regulated as well,

You do not need to get the majority of your calories from the fat with the Atkins diet – you simply limit your carbohydrates. Many people naturally turn to proteins such as meat or fish over fats when they reduce carbohydrates, like a butter stick. "That's why you hear people say that high protein is a keto diet," she said.

Atkins' adjusted diet is a cross between the two. You restrict carbohydrates and cannot enjoy protein. Fats, though not as much as with the traditional ketogenic diet, is promoted.

You're still ready to eat what you can and cannot eat, so to speak. First, let's talk about what a ketogenic diet is.

Any diet forces the body into a ketosis process. This is the mechanism in which fats are absorbed by energy rather than by carbohydrates. When done properly, the keto diet needs the dietitian to eat high quantities of fats, moderate quantities of protein and very low quantities of carbs.

The bodies normally turn carbohydrates in the traditional diet into glucose, which is sent throughout the body as a source of energy. In the keto diet, we get ketosis by which our carbohydrates which causes our liver to break down fatty cells into fatty acids and ketones to be used as energy.

Ketogenic originates from the ketones formed naturally in the body. These are created by the use of fat as energy.

We eat mainly protein, carbohydrates and some fat in a normal or conventional diet. The additional fat is stored.

You eat more fats, very few carbohydrates, and just enough protein for growth in a ketogenic diet.

When the body produces ketones, fat is used to produce energy. The body produces glucose or blood sugar when you eat carbohydrates.

The body enters a ketosis state when it is on the keto diet. Ketosis is a state of energy in which the body uses alternative fuel to supply energy. Instead of using carbohydrates for fuel, it starts to burn fat.

If you eat a very low level of carbohydrates, you get ketosis which depends on the plan and stage you follow. It's normally 20 grams a day, to start with. Your diet is primarily fat, carbohydrates and green vegetables.

Like many low-carb diets, the keto diet is not a new fad. Due to the launch of Dr Atkins New Diet Movement in the 1990s, Dr Robert Atkins became more popular in recent years. It's easy to follow a very effective plan without feeling hungry or craving.

The ability to lose weight without exercise is another reason for its popularity. Those who are severely obese with disabilities or accidents that hinder regular exercises of any kind will find the diet beneficial in weight loss.

CHAPTER 2:

BENEFITS AND RISKS OF THE DIET FOR AFTER 50

There are many ways in which ketosis and the use of safe ketogenic diets are frequently discussed by older people today: Resistance to insulin: many senior citizens in our community struggle with insulin-related disorders such as diabetes and overweight. It is important because diabetes can lead to vision loss, kidney failure and more. Osteoporosis, in which decreased osteoporosis contributes to fragility and fragility of the bones, is one of the most common disorders in older men and women.

More calcium is clearly not the solution, as the USDA advises, via regular intakes of milk products.

That is because the osteoporosis countries continue to have the highest milk intake levels.

Far better than overloading a single macronutrient (calcium), the focus is on a keto diet that is low in toxic substances that impair absorption and is abundant in all micronutrients.

Inflammation: Ageing causes more suffering from younger injuries or joint issues such as arthritis for many individuals.

Being involved in ketosis can lead to reducing the development of substances called cytokines which can help with inflammation.

Nutrient deficiencies: Older adults appear to have higher nutrient deficiencies such as:

- Iron: deficiency can lead to brain nebula and tiredness
- Vitamin B12: deficiency can be responsible for neurological disorders such as dementia
- Fats: deficiencies can cause cognition, skin, and vision and vitamin problems
- Vitamin D: a deficiency in old adults, causes cognitive decline, raises the risk of heart disease and also encourages the risk of cancer.

The high-quality sources of animal protein in the ketogenic diet will easily compensate for these essential nutrients' excellent sources.

KETOGENIC DIETS CAN HELP YOU LOSE WEIGHT

A ketogenic diet is a successful way of losing weight and reducing disease risk factors.

Research indicates that the ketogenic diet is much preferable to the low-fat diet, which is often recommended.

Moreover, the diet is so full that you can lose weight without counting calories or tracking the consumption of food.

For one study, people who have a ketogenic diet lose 2, 2 times as much weight as people who have a low-fat calorie diet. The cholesterol levels of triglycerides and HDL have increased.

Another research showed that people on the ketogenic diet lose three times the weight of the diet prescribed by Diabetes Great Britain.

There are many reasons that a ketogenic diet is preferable to a fat diet, including the increased consumption of protein that provides other benefits.

Increased ketones, lower blood sugar levels and improved response to insulin may also play a crucial role.

CONTROLLING BLOOD SUGAR

The correlation between low blood sugar and conditions related to brain disorders such as Alzheimer's disease, diabetes, and Parkinson's disease has been addressed. Some factors that can support Alzheimer's disease include:

An excess intake of carbohydrates in the ketogenic diet, particularly of fructose.

A reduction of dietary fats and the excess and health of cholesterol on the ketogenic diet

Oxidative stress that protects against ketosis

Following a ketogenic diet to regulate blood sugar and boost nutrition will help not only enhance insulin reaction but also protect you against age memory issues.

WHAT TO KEEP IN MIND WHEN CREATING YOUR KETOGENIC MEAL PLAN

When you wanted to try the keto diet, you would have to adhere to the eating plan guidelines. Approximately 60 to 80 percent of the calories are fats. She says you should eat foods, fats, and oils, and very few non-tarchy plants. (It is different from the conventional low carbon diet since fewer carbohydrates are allowed in the keto diet.)

The remaining calories in the keto diet are extracted from protein — approximately 1 gram (g)/kg, which means that a woman of 140 pounds requires about 64 g of total protein. As for carbs, "Each body is different, but with net carbs between 20 and 50 g per day, most people sustain ketosis," said Mattinson. She states that total carbohydrates minus fiber are equal to net carbs.

One thing I must recall: "It's easy to get ketosis kicked off," Mattinson says. That means, if you eat something as small as a portion of blueberry, your body could transform to fuel and not fat burning carbohydrates.

IMPORTANCE OF KETO FOR AGING

Keto foods have a high amount of calorie content. It is significant because the basal metabolic rate (the number of calories needed daily to survive) is lower for seniors, but the same number of nutrients they still need as younger people. An individual over the age of 65 can survive on fast food a lot harder than a teen or 20-something whose body remains resilient. This makes it even more important for older people to consume health-care and disease-fighting food. It can literally mean the difference between the greatest happiness or suffering and misery in the golden years. Seniors must also consume healthier diets by limiting the use of "empty calories" in sugars or foods high in anti-nutrients, such as whole grains, and increasing their nutritional balance of fats and proteins.

Furthermore, a lot of the food preferred by the elderly (or delivered in clinics or hospitals) is highly processed and low in nutrients such as white bread, pulp, pancakes, etc. It is very clear that the government's high-carb diet is not ideal for helping our seniors and their long-term wellbeing. A diet low in carbohydrates and high in plant and animal fats are much healthier for encouraging improved sensitivity to insulin, less cognitive impairments and better overall health.

CHAPTER 3:

KETOSIS FOR LONGEVITY

It's never a bad thing to boost your chances of feeling and to work well for the rest of your life, no matter what our generation. It is never too late to try to do better, even though the earlier we arrive, the greater the likelihood of disease prevention. Also, for those who have not handled their bodies as well as they can for several years, ketosis for older people has the ability to repair such damage.

CAN WE LIVE LONGER IN KETOSIS?

This is a worth exploring issue, particularly as people live longer but suffer from often dietary- and lifestyle-related illnesses. Here are some of the current research on the potential for longevity ketosis:

KETOSIS AND MITOCHONDRIA

One of the longevity hypotheses is that the secret to longer lives is to handle our mitochondria as they are responsible for the production of energy in our cells. Ketosis is considered to have extremely beneficial effects on the mitochondrial function:

- Increased antioxidant levels in mitochondria.
- Increase the number of mitochondria in hippocampus neurons in rats, which is essential for normal brain function.
- Decreasing the number of reactive oxygen species that damage cell structures of mitochondria in high quantities.

KETOSIS AND AGING-RELATED DISEASE

Ageing diseases clearly have a major impact on survival, which is why it is important to look at the effect of ketosis on these diseases. Below are several ways in which ketones have shown possible benefits:

Acetoacetate cetones have shown to prevent neurotoxicity in brain cells in mouse models.

A small study found that patients with Parkinson's disease had good outcomes following a ketogenic diet for 28 days. Another small study showed that ketones orally administered to adults with Alzheimer's disease improved cognition every day in 90 days. Large studies are needed on humans, but these findings may be useful for protecting us from the deterioration that is seen in many of our people as they age.

LOW-CARB FOR LONGEVITY

We know that a diet full of high-quality protein, colourful vegetables and healthy fats, with low carbon and sugar intake antioxidants, is a powerful way to promote our health. Although not specific to ketosis, the simply low-carbon and complete nutritional quality of the ketogenic diet offers us a number of benefits that can protect us against common food conditions, including cardiac diseases, diabetes and obesity. Elders without these worries reduces the possibility of dying from them, which is, of course, perfect for the entire lifetime.

CALORIE RESTRICTION

Research has also shown that the ketogenic diet has the ability to slow down the effects of ageing. Carbohydrate metabolism can cause aspects of the aging process, whereas the calorie restriction that causes the body to consume free fatty acids can slow the aging process. Also, with regard to the calorie reduction of ant-ageing, ketosis is an effective way of consuming less food in general because of our high degree of satisfaction with fats and good-quality proteins.

KETOSIS FOR MENTAL LONGEVITY

Mental health is an important part of living longer and more satisfying, especially with worsening cognitive disorders like Alzheimer's and dementia, which are so prevalent in aging populations today.

Research has shown that ketogenic diets can have protective effects, including:

Ketosis for neurodegenerative diseases: After a ketogenic diet, both factors can help minimize neurodegenerative and age-related cognitive disorders, which can have a significant effect on the quality of life as we grow older. Beta-hydroxybutyrate protective effects:

Ketone body beta-hydroxybutyrate can provide protective protection against Parkinson's and Alzheimer's diseases. Beta-hydroxybutyrate plays an important function in the health of the brain. Cognitive impairment ketosis: ketosis has been shown to benefit adults with Alzheimer's memory impairment, providing an alternative fuel source to glucose.

Besides the potential of ketosis for beneficial effects on survival, it is also worth remembering how diets equate most people today to the traditional American Standard Diet (SAD).

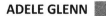

THE KETOGENIC DIET VS WESTERN DIET AND AGING

Research on ketosis and anti-aging, as you can see, promises that the ketogenic diet will support longevity. The downside is that the bulk of ketosis and ketogenic dietary work so far were done in animal studies. This is understandable because longevity studies in ketosis on humans take a very long time to check their effects reliably on normal human ageing.

That said, ketogenic diets certainly don't appear to damage our longevity chances by taking into account all the advantages they can bring, especially in comparison to what is eaten in the majority of the Western world: large quantities of refined carbohydrates, sugars and other packaged foods, which give little or no nutritional quality. The long-term harm done by this way of eating is much more significant. It is very clear to tell.

CHAPTER 4:

FOODS TO AVOID ON THE DIET

Every food high in carbohydrates should be reduced. Here is a list of foods for a ketogenic diet to be reduced or eliminated:
Fruit: All fruit, except small portions of berries like strawberries.
Alcohol: Because of its carb, several alcoholic drinks will throw you out of the ketosis.
Sugar-free diet foods: They are often high in sugar alcohols, which in some cases can affect ketone levels. These foods are also extensively processed.
Beans or legumes: Peas, kidney beans, lentils, chickpeas, etc.
Grains or starches: Wheat-based products, rice, pasta, cereal, etc.
Low-fat or diet products: These are highly processed and often high in carbs.
Some condiments or sauces: These often contain sugar and unhealthy fat.
Root vegetables and tubers: Potatoes, sweet potatoes, carrots, parsnips, etc.
Sugary foods: Soda, fruit juice, smoothies, cake, ice cream, candy, etc.
Unhealthy fats: Limit your intake of processed vegetable oils, mayonnaise, etc.
Remove carbohydrates such as wheat, vegetables, legumes, rice, potatoes, sweets, milk, and most fruits.

CHAPTER 5:

FOODS TO EAT ON THE DIET

Wonder what's in a keto diet — and what doesn't? "It is so important to know what foods you're going to consume and how to add more fats to your diet before you start."

PROTEIN

Liberally: (That said, ketogenic diets are not rich in protein and are based on fat and should be moderately eaten.)

Grass-fed beef

Fish, especially fatty fish, like salmon

Dark meat chicken

Occasionally: Bacon

Low-fat proteins such as shrimp and skinless chicken breast. They are perfect for your keto diet but add a sauce to your meal instead of eating straight.

Never: Marinatedmeatdeep in sugary sauces

Chicken nuggets or fishnuggets

OIL AND FAT

- Heavy cream
- Butter
- Coconut oil
- Avocado oil
- Olive oil

Reduce your intake, which you need to do conveniently in order to avoid processed foods, frequently contained in them.

- Safflower oil
- Corn oil
- Sunflower oil

Never:

- Margarine
- Artificial trans fats

FRUITS AND VEGGIES

- Celery
- Asparagus
- Avocado
- Leafy greens, like spinach and arugula

Occasionally: There are all great options, but these carbs do have to be counted.

- Eggplant
- Leeks
- Spaghetti squash

Never:

- Raisins
- Potatoes
- Corn

Nuts and Seeds
- Flaxseed and chia seeds
- Walnuts
- Almonds

Occasionally:
- Pistachios
- Cashews
- almond or peanut butter

Never:
- Chocolate-covered nuts
- Trail mixes with dried fruit
- Sweetened nut or seed butters

Dairy Products
- Feta cheese
- Cheddar cheese
- Blue cheese

Occasionally:
- Full-fat ricotta cheese
- Full-fat cottage cheese
- Full-fat plain Greek yoghurt

Never:
- Ice cream
- Sweetened nonfat yoghurt
- Milk

Sweeteners
Occasionally:
- Erythritol
- Xylitol
- Stevia

Never:
- White and brown sugars
- Maple syrup
- Agave
- Honey

Condiments and Sauces
- Mayonnaise (no sugar)
- Guacamole
- Lemon butter sauce

Occasionally:
- Tomato sauce (no sugar version)
- Balsamic vinegar
- Raw garlic

Never:
- Ketchup
- Barbecue sauce
- Honey mustard

DRINKS

- Plain tea
- Almond milk
- Water
- Bone broth

Occasionally:

- Diet soda
- Unsweetened carbonated water
- Zero-calorie drinks
- Black coffee

Never:

- Fruit juice
- Lemonade
- Soda

HERBS AND SPICES

All herbs and spices fit into a keto diet, but Mancinelli recommends that you count the carb if you use large amounts.

- Thyme, oregano, paprika, and cayenne
- Salt (salt foods to taste)
- Pepper

Occasionally: These are all excellent options, but they include some carbs.

- Onion powder
- Ground ginger
- Garlic powder

Never:

Herbs and spices are usually all right to be used to add flavour to food in limited quantities.

SUPPLEMENTS

- Multivitamin
- Fibre

Optional: This helps you make ketones easier, but Mancinelli says she doesn't have an opinion to suggest whether you take them or not.

- Exogenous ketones
- MCT oil

DETAILED KETOGENIC DIET FOOD LIST TO FOLLOW

The ketogenic diet has recently become very common.

Evidence has shown the efficacy of a very low-carbon, high-fat diet for weight loss, diabetes and epilepsy.

It is also early evidence that certain cancers, Alzheimer's disease, and other disorders may also benefit.

A ketogenic diet typically limits carbohydrates to 20-50 g / day.

While this can be difficult, many healthy foods can easily be used to eat this way.

Healthy foods to eat on a ketogenic diet are available here.

1. Seafood

Fish and mushrooms are particularly keto-friendly foods. The salmon and other fish are abundant, although nearly free of oil, in B vitamins, potassium and selenium.

The carbs in different shellfish types vary, however.

For example, while shrimp and most crabs do not contain carbon, there are other types of coquillages.

Although these shellfish can still be used in a ketogenic diet, it is crucial to take these carbs into consideration when you seek to remain within a narrow range.

Here are the carbohydrates for 3.5-ounce portions of some common types of shellfish:

- Octopus: 4 grams
- Oysters: 4 grams
- Clams: 5 grams
- Mussels: 7 grams
- Squid: 3 grams

Salmon, sardines, mackerel, and other fatty fish are very rich in omega-3 fats that have been shown to decrease insulin levels and to improve overweight and obese sensitivity to insulin.

Moreover, a decreased risk of disease and enhanced mental health were correlated with the daily consumption of fish.

In order to eat at least two servings of seafood regularly.

Many seafood types are carbon-free or very low in carbs. Even healthy sources of vitamins, minerals and omega-3s are fish and shellfish.

2. Low-Carb Vegetables

Non-starchy vegetables have low calories and carbohydrates but are high in many nutrients, including vitamin C and minerals.

Vegetables and other plants contain fiber that does not digest and enter the body as other carbs do.

Look at your digestible (or net) carb count, which is total carbs less fiber.

Most plants contain very few net carbohydrates. But you could consume a serving of "starchy" vegetables such as potatoes, yams or beets for the day.

For nonstarchy vegetables, the net carb count ranges from 1 gram for 1 cup of raw spinach to 8 grams for 1 cup of cooked Brussels sprouts.

Vegetables also contain antioxidants to prevent free radicals, which are unstable molecules that can damage the cells.

Moreover, cruciferous plants such as kale, broccoli and cauliflower have been associated with reduced risk of cancer and heart disease.

Low-carbon vegetables make a big substitute for higher-carbon foods.

For example, cauliflower can be used to imitate rice or mashed potatoes, "zoodles" can be produced from courgettes and spaghetti squash is a natural replacement to spaghetti.

Net carbs are between 1–8 grams per cup in non-starchy vegetables.

Vegetables are healthy, flexible and can lead to reducing disease risk.

3. Cheese

Both nutritious and delicious is cheese.

Hundreds of kinds of cheese exist.

Fortunately, they are all very small in carbs and fat, making them quite good for a ketogenic diet.

One ounce of cheddar cheese (28 grams) contains 1 gram of carbohydrate and 7 grams of protein and 20 percent of calcium RDI.

Cheese is high in saturated fat, but the risk of heart disease has not been shown to increase.

In addition, some studies indicate that cheese can protect against cardiovascular disease.

Cheese also includes conjugated linoleic acid, a fat-related to loss of weight and changes in the structure of the body. Furthermore, eating cheese frequently will help reduce the loss of muscle weight and strength with aging.

In a 12-week study of old adults, people who drank 7 ounces (210 grams) of ricotta daily had an increase in muscle mass and muscular strength during the test.

Cheese is high in protein, calcium and protective fatty acids and also has a low amount of carbohydrate.

4. Avocados

Avocados are amazingly well.

3.5 ounces (100 g), or about half a medium avocado, contain 9 grams of carbohydrates.

Seven of these are fiber, however, and thus their net carbon count is just 2 grams.

Avocados are rich in many vitamins and minerals, including potassium. Many people do not get enough of a significant mineral.

In addition, a higher intake of potassium can make the transition to a ketogenic diet easier.

Avocados can also help to boost the level of cholesterol and triglyceride.

In one study, when people a diet high in avocados, "bad" LDL cholesterol and triglycerides were 22 percent lower and "good" HDL cholesterol 11 percent higher.

Avocados contain 2 grams per serving of net carbs and are high in fiber and a number of nutrients including potassium.

They can also improve heart safety markers.

5. Meat and Poultry

Meat and poultry in a ketogenic diet are considered essential food.

No carbs and B vitamins and several minerals are rich in fresh meat and poultry, including potassium, selenium and zinc.

These are also an important source of high-quality protein that has been tested in a low-carb diet to help maintain muscle mass.

An elderly woman study found that consuming high-fat diets in fatty meat led to 8 percent higher HDL cholesterol levels than using a low-fat high-carb diet.

If possible, it is best to choose grass-fed poultry.

It's because grass-driven animals produce meat with higher omega-3-fat, linoleic acid conjugated, and antioxidants than animal-driven meat. Fleece and poultry contain no carbohydrates and are rich in high-quality protein and other nutrients.

The healthiest alternative is grass-fed beef.

6. Eggs

Eggs are one of the most nutritious and versatile foods in the world.

Eggs have less than 1 gram of carbohydrates and less than 6 gram of protein in one large egg and are thus suitable for a ketogenic lifestyle.

Furthermore, eggs have been shown to activate hormones that increase fullness sensations and keep blood sugar levels steady, resulting in lower intakes of calories for up to 24 hours.

The whole of the egg should be consumed because much of the nutrients in an egg are stored in the yolk. It includes lutein and zeaxanthin, antioxidants that protect the protection of the body.

While egg yolks are high in cholesterol, their consumption in most people does not increase blood cholesterol.

Yes, eggs appear to alter the shape of LDL so as to reduce the risk of cardiovascular disease.

Eggs contain less than 1 gram of carbs and can help you preserve them for hours.

These are also rich in many nutrients and can protect the health of the eye and of the heart.

7. Coconut Oil

Coconut oil has unique features that make it suitable for a ketogenic diet.

It contains triglycerides in the medium-chain (MCTs). In comparison to long-chain fats, MCTs are taken up directly by the liver and converted into ketones or used as a strong energy source.

Indeed, coconut oil was used to increase the levels of ketone in people with Alzheimer's disease and other brain and nervous system disorders.

Lauric acid, a slightly longer chain fat, is the main fatty acid in cocoa oil. Cocoside oil blends of MCTs and lauric acid have been proposed to encourage a safe degree of ketosis.

Moreover, cocoa oil can assist obese adults in losing weight and fat.

In one study, men who eat two tablespoons (30 ml) of coconut oil a day lost on average 1 inch (2.5 cm), without any other changes in their diet.

Cocoon oil is rich in MCTs, which can improve the production of ketone.

It may also increase the metabolic rate and encourage weight and abdominal fat loss.

8. Plain Greek Yogurt and Cottage Cheese

Plain Greek yogurt and cottage cheese are high-protein, nutritious food.

These can also have some carbohydrates in a ketogenic lifestyle.

Five ounces (150 grams) of plain Greek yogurt contains five grams of carbs and eleven grams of protein.

Cottage cheese contains 5 grams of carbohydrates and 18 grams of protein.

Yoghurt and cottage cheese have been demonstrated to suppress hunger and to promote fullness feelings

Whether you make a tasty snack on your own.

Nevertheless, they can also be mixed with chopped nuts, cinnamon and optional sugar-free sweeteners to handle them quickly and easily.

Both plain and cottage yogurt contain 5 grams of carbohydrate per serving.

Research has shown that they contribute to decreased appetite and to fullness.

9. Olive Oil

Olive oil gives your heart impressive benefits.

It is high in oleic acid, a monounsaturated fat found to lower the risk factors of heart disease in many studies. Extra virgin olive oil, also known as phenols, is high in antioxidants.

These compounds further protect cardiac health by reducing inflammation and improving the function of the artery.

Olive oil contains no carbohydrates as a pure source of fat. It is a perfect basis for balanced mayonnaise and salad dressings. As it is not as stable as saturated fats at high temperatures, olive oil can be used for cooking at low temperatures or added to food after it is cooked.

Olive oil can be found online.

Extra-virgin olive oil is high in monounsaturated and antioxidant heart-healthy fats.

It is ideal for dressings for salads, mayonnaise and cooked foods.

10. Nuts and Seeds

Nuts and seeds are balanced foods with high fat and low carbon content. Reduced risk of heart disease, other cancers, depression and other chronic diseases were correlated with daily nut intake. In fact, nuts and seeds are rich in fibre, meaning you can feel full and eat fewer calories. Although all nuts and seeds are low in net carbohydrates, the quantities vary greatly from one type to another. Here are the 1 ounce (28 grams) carb numbers for some common nuts and seeds:

- Cashews: 8 grams net carbs (9 grams total carbs)
- Almonds: 3 grams net carbs (6 grams total carbs)
- Brazil nuts: 1 gram net carbs (3 grams total carbs)Pistachios: 5 grams net carbs (8 grams total carbs)
- Walnuts: 2 grams net carbs (4 grams total carbs)

- Chia seeds: 1 gram net carbs (12 grams total carbs)
- Flaxseeds: 0 grams net carbs (8 grams total carbs)
- Macadamia nuts: 2 grams net carbs (4 grams total carbs)
- Pecans: 1 gram net carbs (4 grams total carbs)
- Pumpkin seeds: 4 grams net carbs (5 grams total carbs)
- Sesame seeds: 3 grams net carbs (7 grams total carbs)

Nuts and seeds are cardiovascular, fibre-rich, and can help in healthy ageing. They have 0–8 grams per ounce of net carbon.

11. Berries

Many fruits are too large for a ketogenic diet in carbs, but berries are an exception.

Beers are low in carbohydrates and high in antioxidants.

Raspberries and blackberries also produce as much fibre as digestible carbs.

Such small fruits are filled with antioxidants associated with inflammation reduction and disease prevention.

Here are the carb counts for certain berries for 3.5 ounces (100 grams):

- Blueberries: 12 grams net carbs (14 grams total carbs)
- Strawberries: 6 grams net carbs (8 grams total carbs)
- Blackberries: 5 grams net carbs (10 grams total carbs)
- Raspberries: 6 grams net carbs (12 grams total carbs)

Berriesare rich in nutrients that can reduce disease risk.

They supply 5–12 grams net carbs per 3.5-ounce part.

12. Butter and Cream

Butter and cream are healthy fats for a ketogenic diet.

Everyone only contains trace amounts of carbs per serving.

Butter and cream have been known to cause or lead to heart disease for many years because of their high levels of saturated fat. However, several broad studies have shown that saturated fat is not associated with heart disease for most people.

In addition, some studies show that moderate consumption of fatty milk can reduce the risk of heart attack and stroke.

Butter and cream are abundant, like other fatty milk products, in conjugated linoleic acid, the fatty acid that may contribute to fat loss.

Butter and cream are nearly carbon-free and tend to have a moderately consumed neutral or positive impact on heart health.

13. Shirataki Noodles

Shirataki noodles are an excellent supplement to a ketogenic diet. They can be searched online.

These contain less than 1 gram of carbs and five calories per serving, mostly because it is water.

These noodles are in reality made from a viscous fibre called glucomannan which can absorb its weight up to 50 times in water.

Viscous fiber is a gel which slows the movement of food through your digestive tract. It will help reduce appetite and blood sugar spikes, which helps to control weight loss and diabetes.

Shirataki noodles come in various kinds, rice, fettuccine and linguine included. These can be replaced in all forms of recipes by standard noodles.

Shirataki noodles contain less than 1 gram per serving of carbs. A viscous fiber helps ease the flow of food through the digestive tract, which encourages blood sugar levels and completeness.

14. Olives

Only in solid form do olives have the same health benefits as olive oil. The key antioxidant found in olives, oleuropein has anti-inflammatory properties and can protect against damage to your cells. Studies also say that olive intake can help prevent bone loss and lower blood pressure. Because of their size, the olives differ in carb content. However, half of their carbohydrates come from fiber, so they have a low digestible carb content. A one-ounce portion of olive (28-gram) contains 2 grams of total carbs and 1 gram of fiber. This results in a net carb count of 1 gram, depending on the size, for 7 to 10 olives.

Olives are rich in antioxidants that can protect the health of the heart and body. They contain 1 grams net carbohydrates per ounce.

15. Unsweetened Coffee and Tea

Coffee and tea are unbelievably healthy and carb-free.

It contains caffeine, which enhances your metabolism and your physical health, alertness and mood.

In fact, coffee and tea consumers have shown that the risk of diabetes is significantly reduced. In addition, those who drink the highest amount of coffee and tea are at the lowest risk for diabetes.

Heavy cream is nice to add to coffee or tea but stay away from "hot" coffee and tea lattes. These are usually made from non-fat milk and have high-carbon flavours.

No carbohydrates in unsweetened coffee and tea will help improve your metabolic and physical and mental health. You may also reduce diabetes risk.

16. Dark Chocolate and Cocoa Powder

Dark chocolate and cocoa are delicious antioxidant sources.

In reality, cacao was known as "superfruit," because it has at least as much antioxidant activity as any other fruit, like blueberries and acai berries.

Dark chocolate contains flavanols that can help lower blood pressure and keep the arteries safe, which can reduce the risk of heart disease.

Surprisingly, chocolate can be used in the ketogenic diet. However, choosing dark chocolate that contains at least 70% of the cocoa solids, preferably more, is essential.

One ounce (28 grams) of unsweetened chocolate has 3 grams of net carbohydrate (100% cocoa). The same volume of 70-85% dark chocolate contains up to 10 g net carbohydrates.

Dark chocolate contains 3–10 grams per ounce of net carbohydrates, is rich in antioxidants and can reduce the risk of cardiac disease.

KETOGENIC SNACK OPTIONS

Snacking between meals will help reduce hunger and keep you up with a ketogenic diet.

Since the ketogenic diet is so full, only one or two snacks a day may be needed depending on the level of your operation.

Here are some good, easy to use snacks:

- Cheese roll-ups
- Parmesan crisps
- Guacamole with low-carb veggies
- Hard-boiled eggs
- Coconut chips
- Almonds and cheddar cheese
- Kale chips
- Olives and sliced salami
- Celery and peppers with herbed cream cheese dip
- Trail mix made with unsweetened coconut, nuts and seeds
- Berries with heavy whipping cream
- Jerky
- Macadamia nuts
- Greens with high-fat dressing and avocado
- Keto smoothie made with coconut milk, cocoa and avocado
- Avocado cocoa mousse

Although these keto snacks can maintain their fullness between meals, they can also help to increase the weight if you snack too much all day long.

It's important to eat the right amount of calories according to your level of activity, weight loss target, age and gender.

Keto-friendly snacks should be fatty, low in protein, and low in carbs. Enhance your fibre intake by snacking with a fat dipping sauce on sliced, low-carb vegetables.

CHAPTER 6:

KETO DIET TIPS

magine you have practised the Keto diet for some time, and you find it impossible to stick to guidelines unexpectedly. You want to add a few carbs. Or you're sick of the same old food. Or that you don't get any encouragement from those around you.

Here are some tips to help you stick to the diet.

GET SUPPORT.

Join online forums and communities in which most practice the same diet. Encourage friends and family to indulge in the ketogenic diet.

FOCUS ON THE GOOD THINGS.

Concentrate on what you have already done. Do you feel more vigorous? Has your night got better? How do you feel relative to your Keto diet before you began?

GET BACK ON IF YOU FALL OFF.

Do not give up if you fall and eat a slice of cake or drink a beer. It is naive to expect that you won't often slip into temptation. The aim is to return to a healthier option. However, note that the body suffers from ketosis when you eat a certain amount of carbohydrates. And it takes you a few days to get back into it.

BE PREPARED.

Get your materials, books, and foods before you start your diet. Remove your cupboard from everything you shouldn't eat, so you are less likely to be tented.

SET UP AN ACCOUNTABILITY SYSTEM.

Have anyone to keep you accountable for adhering to the program.

ADD EXERCISE.

Add a high-intensity workout schedule after the first month. It can be as easy as a fast walk. Add weight training once a week to help lose fat.

WHEN EXERCISING, YOU MAY NEED TO CHANGE YOUR KETO DIET TO A TARGETED OR CYCLICAL PLAN.

The cyclic ketogenic diet is used to incorporate a carbohydrate on weekends and after a regular keto diet throughout the week. A targeted ketogenic diet plan requires you to eat some extra carbs before you work out.

BE PATIENT AND DON'T CHEAT.

It takes time to start burning fat and get into ketosis. Keep on it and remain consistent. Don't every day measure yourself? Due to water intake and absorption, weight varies from 2 to 4 pounds every day.

TRACK YOUR PROGRESS AND EATING HABITS.

Using a newspaper, an electronic notepad or a smartphone device. Measure what you eat and write it down. Keep track of the consumption of calories, fat, protein and carbohydrate.

As you can see, on this trip, you're not alone. If you feel like leaving, there are many ways to get help. The first step is to be careful and compliant with the strategy. It is simpler and the more support and accountability you have, the more likely you are to stick it out.

MEASURING PROGRESS AND YOUR RESULTS

No doubt one of the most motivating things about weight loss is that you can see and measure your results. I say, in the mirror, you look at yourself, and your clothes get looser.

Can you imagine how huge it feels? That's great feeling to be certain. But you really need to measure your progress to make sure the keto diet works. There are various ways to monitor your success.

One way is by measuring ketosis.

The way this is done is by measuring the cells' bi-product ketones released from the body. Sweat and urine come out with your breath. Self-testing urine strips to test your urine allow you to see when your body is ketosis first, and you stay ketosis. The strips are colour-neutral and during ketosis change to shades of light pink to deep purple. The darker the light, the more you burn. You should buy a blood ketone meter later.

One alternative is a full blood chemistry check before you start and then begin the diet for one month. It shows improvements in cholesterol and blood sugar.

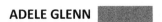

You should calculate weight loss once a week, ideally simultaneously. You will probably see a big improvement within the first week. Yet don't be fooled. Don't be fooled. Some of them will be a lack of weight, but others will also be water loss.

As a way to track weight loss, measure yourself. You can gain weight from lean muscle mass while you focus on your diet. To assess your weight loss, you will see if you lose inches.

Measuring and tracking your weight loss while on the ketogenic diet is a simple process that will allow you to stay motivated.

CHAPTER 7:

KETO DIET SHOPPING LIST

Many fresh foods, healthy fats and proteins will form part of a well-rounded ketogenic diet. If you select a combination of both fresh and frozen items, you will be able to supply keto-friendly fruit and vegetables to be added to your recipe. The following is a basic ketogenic shopping list that will lead you through the food corridors:

Meat and poultry: Beef, chicken, turkey and pork (choose organic, pasture-raised options whenever possible).

Fish: Fatty fish like salmon, sardines, mackerel and herring are best.

Shellfish: Oysters, shrimp and scallops.

Eggs: Purchase omega-3-enriched or pastured eggs whenever possible.

Full-fat dairy: Unsweetened yoghurt, butter, heavy cream and sour cream.

Oils: Coconut and avocado oils.

Avocados: Buy a mixture of ripe and unripe avocados so that your supply will last.

Cheese: Brie, cream cheese, cheddar and goat cheese.

Frozen or fresh berries: Blueberries, raspberries, blackberries. Nuts: Macadamia nuts, almonds, pecans, pistachios. Seeds: Pumpkin seeds, sunflower seeds, chia seeds. Nut butter: Almond butter, peanut butter. Fresh or frozen low-carb vegetables: Mushrooms, cauliflower, broccoli, greens, peppers, onions and tomatoes. Condiments: Sea salt, pepper, salsa, herbs, garlic, vinegar, mustard, olives and spices.

It is also worth planning your meals beforehand and filling your cart with the ingredients needed for healthy dishes worth a few days. In addition, it can help to avoid tempting, unhealthy food by sticking to a shopping list.

A shopping list will help you determine which food suits your ketogenic meal plan. Load your cart with meat, fish, eggs, fatty veggies and healthy fats.

CHAPTER 8:

21 DAYS MEAL PLAN

The keto diet is usually very low in carbohydrates, high in fat and mild in protein. When a ketogenic diet is followed, carbs are usually lower than 50 grams a day, although there are stricter and looser variations of the diet. The bulk of cut carbs will be substituted by fats and about 75% of the overall calorie intake.

Proteins will account for approximately 20%, while carbohydrates are typically limited to 5%.

This carb reduction causes the body to rely on fat instead of glucose – the cycle called ketosis – for its key energy source. While your body uses ketones – molecules formed in the liver from fat when glucose is reduced – as an alternative source of fuel during ketosis.

While fat is often avoided due to its high-calorie content, evidence shows that ketogenic diets are far more effective than low-fat diets in promoting weight loss. Keto diets also reduce hunger and improve satiety, which can be beneficial in weight loss. The ketogenic diet is based on a very low carbon routine. Carbs are typically reduced to less than 50 grams a day and are primarily supplemented with fat and moderate quantities of protein. It may seem daunting to turn to a ketogenic diet, but it doesn't have to be difficult. You will concentrate on reducing carbohydrates while rising food and snacks' fat and protein content. Carbs must be limited to enter and stay in a ketosis state. Although some individuals can only achieve ketosis by eating fewer than 20 grams of carbs a day, some can thrive with much higher carbon intakes.

In general, the sooner you enter and remain in ketosis, the lower your carbohydrate intake.

That is why it is the safest way to effectively lose weight in a ketogenic diet to stick to keto-friendly foods and avoid carbohydrates.

KETO MENU FOR 3 WEEKS

Less than 50 grams of total carbs per day are included in the following section. As described above, some people can still have to may carbohydrates to achieve ketosis.

Below is a general one-week ketogenic menu, which can be modified according to each dietary requirement.

WEEK 1

MONDAY

BREAKFAST
Scrambled eggs
Butter plus eggs are the perfect breakfast for you. Start your day right with our especially buttery version of this classic breakfast. Up in minutes! Out in minutes!
Ingredients
- 1 oz. butter
- Two eggs
- salt and pepper

INSTRUCTIONS
Crack the eggs in a small bowl and use a bucket to whisk them with salt and pepper.
Melt the butter over medium heat in a non-stick skillet. Monitor attentively — butter shouldn't become brown!
Place the eggs into the saucepan and remove for 1–2 minutes, until fluffy and fried, as you like. Remember that even though you put it on your plate, the eggs will still be fried.

LUNCH
Keto Asian beef salad
Gingery and savoury with a spicy kick. Hearty red meat of creamy goodness with sesame. All this, keto, and a healthy boot salad?? Can you see where we're going?

INGREDIENTS
- Sesame mayonnaise

- ¾ cup mayonnaise
- 1 tsp.Sesame oil
- ½ tbsp. lime juice
- salt and pepper
- Beef
- 1 tbsp. olive oil
- 1 tbsp. fish sauce
- 1 tbsp. grated fresh ginger
- 1 tsp. chilli flakes
- 2/3 lb.rib-eye steaks
- Salad
- 3 oz. cherry tomatoes
- 2 oz. cucumber
- 3 oz. lettuce
- ½ red onion
- fresh cilantro
- 1 tsp. sesame seeds
- Two scallions

INSTRUCTIONS

By mixing mayonnaise with sesame oil and lime juice, prepare the mayonnaise sesame. Salt and pepper season. Pack. Set aside. Set aside. Mix all-beef marinade ingredients and pour into a plastic container. Remove the beef and marinate at room temperature for 15 minutes or more. Cut all vegetables into bite bits, except the scallions. Split into two boards. Over medium heat, heat a medium frying pan. Add sesame to the pan and toast for a few minutes, or until lightly browned and fragrant. Set aside. Set aside. Pat the meat dry with paper towels on both sides. Sear for a minute or two at high heat on each side, then cut down to medium-low heat, cook until beef is medium and then move to a cutting board.

Fry the scallions in the same pot for a minute.

Slice the meat into thin slices across the grain. Place on top of the vegetable beef and scallions.

Add the roasted sesame seeds and serve with a sesame mayonnaise dollop on the side.

DINNER

Chicken saucepan keto with feta and olives

The fluffy, easy to make keto chicken platter is made up of feta cheese, olives, and pesto.

Give it a try, whether you are using low-carb, shopping or your own homemade pesto. You're going to thank your taste buds — and your mates!

Ingredients

- 1½ lbs. boneless chicken thighs or chicken breasts
- salt and pepper
- 2 tbsp. butter or coconut oil
- 5 tbsp. red pesto or green pesto
- 1¼ cups heavy whipping cream
- 3 oz. pitted olives
- 5 oz. feta cheese, diced
- One garlic clove, finely chopped
- For serving
- 5 oz. leafy greens
- 4 tbsp. olive oil
- sea salt and ground black pepper

INSTRUCTIONS

Preheat oven to 200 ° C (400 ° F). Preheat.

Break the chicken into bits in bite-size. Salt and pepper season. Pack.

In a wide skillet add butter or oil and bathe the chicken parts over medium to high heat until golden brown.

Mix pesto and heavy cream in a bowl of store-bought red or green pesto.

Layer the fried chicken pieces with olives, feta and garlic in a baking bowl. Add the mixture of pesto/cream.

Bake 20-30 minutes in the oven, until the dish bubbles around and the edges lightly brown.

TUESDAY

BREAKFAST
Keto cheese roll-ups

This is the world's best, easiest, most keto-lip-smacking technique.
The savoury goodness cannot be avoided!
Ingredients

- 8 oz. cheddar cheese or provolone cheese or Edam cheese, in slices
- 2 oz. butter

INSTRUCTIONS

On a large cutting board position the cheese slices.
Cut the butter with a slicer or cut the bits with a knife very thin.
Cover with butter per cheese slice and roll-up. Serve as a snack.

LUNCH
Keto Caprese omelet

Nice mozzarella, fresh basil, and ripe tomatoes, yes, please! In an omelet — better yet!
This super simple keto dish is perfect for breakfast, lunch or dinner and will surely be a new favourite. So get your saucepan out.
Ingredients

- Six eggs
- salt and pepper
- 1 tbsp. chopped fresh basil or dried basil
- 2 tbsp. olive oil
- 3 oz. cherry tomatoes cut in halves or tomatoes cut in slices
- 5 oz. fresh mozzarella cheese, diced or sliced

INSTRUCTIONS

Crack the eggs in a mixing pot, add salt and black pepper. Whisk well until fully combined with a fork. Incorporate basil and stir. Heat oil in a large pot. For a few minutes, fry the tomatoes. Pour the egg batter over the tomatoes. Before adding the mozzarella cheese, wait until the batter is slightly firm. Reduce heat and leave the omelette in place. Serve immediately and enjoy!

DINNER
Keto meat pie

Keep us pleased with this satisfying cheese-topped masterpiece. Meat pie may be an old age, but now is the time to rediscover its delight.
Ingredients

- Pie crust
- ¾ cup almond flour
- 4 tbsp. sesame seeds
- 4 tbsp. coconut flour
- 1 tbsp. ground psyllium husk powder
- 1 tsp. baking powder
- 1 pinch salt
- 3 tbsp. olive oil or coconut oil, melted
- 1 egg
- 4 tbsp. water

Topping

- 8 oz. cottage cheese
- 7 oz. shredded cheese

Filling

- ½ yellow onion, finely chopped
- 1 garlic clove, finely chopped
- 2 tbsp. butter or olive oil
- 1¼ lbs. ground beef or ground lamb

- 1 tbsp. dried oregano or dried basil
- salt and pepper
- 4 tbsp. tomato paste or ajvar relish
- ½ cup water

INSTRUCTIONS

Preheat oven to 175 ° C (350 ° F). Preheat oven.

Fry onion and garlic over medium heat in butter or olive oil for a few minutes until the onion is tender. Add ground beef and continue to fry. Add basil or oregano. To taste salt and pepper.

Add tomato paste or add to taste. Add water. Add water. Reduce heat and cook for at least 20 minutes. Make the dough for the crust while the meat is simmering.

Mix all the croust ingredients for a few minutes in a food processor until the dough is a ball. You should combine with a fork by hand if you don't have a food processor.

In a well-greased springform pot or deep-greasy piece of parchment paper — 9-10 "(23-25 cm) in diameter — to make removing the pie easier when it is finished. Place the dough in the pot and on the sides. Use a spatula or fingers well grated. When the casserole has been formed, choose the bottom of the crust with a bifurcation.

Bake the crust 10-15 minutes before. Take the meat from the oven and put it in the crust. Combine the cottage cheese with shredded cheese and spread over the pastry.

Bake for 30-40 minutes on the bottom rack or until the pie is golden.

WEDNESDAY

BREAKFAST

Keto frittata with fresh spinach

This stunning dish looks amazing but is incredibly easy to produce! Spinach, cheese, sausages, and vegetables are good for the eyes ... and for the tummy.

Ingredients

- 5 oz. diced bacon or chorizo
- 2 tbsp. butter
- 8 oz. fresh spinach
- 8 eggs
- 1 cup heavy whipping cream
- 5 oz. shredded cheese
- salt and pepper

Instructions

Preheat oven to 175 ° C (350 ° F). Preheat oven. Grate a 9x9 bakery or individual ramekins.

Fry the butter bacon over medium heat to crispy. Attach the spinach and whisk until smooth. Take the heat out of the pot and set aside.

Whisk the eggs and milk and pour in a bakery or ramekins.

Top with bacon, spinach and cheese and put in the middle of the oven. Bake for 25–30 minutes or until golden brown is put on top.

LUNCH

Keto no-noodle chicken soup

Made of healing bone broth, it's warm and comforting, when it is cool outside, if you're fighting a cold or if you're just craving a heart-felt soup!

- Ingredients
- 4 oz. butter
- 2 tbsp. dried minced onion
- 2 celery stalks, chopped
- 6 oz. mushrooms, sliced
- 2 minced garlic cloves
- 8 cups chicken broth
- 1 medium sized carrot, sliced
- 2 tsp. dried parsley
- 1 tsp. salt

- ¼ tsp. ground black pepper
- 1½ rotisserie chicken, shredded
- 5 oz. green cabbage, sliced into strips

INSTRUCTIONS

In a large pot, melt the butter over medium heat.

Into the oven, add dried ointment, chopped celery, sliced champagne and garlic and cook 3-4 minutes.

Add broth, carrot sliced, parsley, salt, and potatoes.

Simmer until tender vegetables.

Add chicken and cooked chicken.

Simmer for a further 8-12 minutes until the chicken "noodles" are tender.

DINNER

Keto Pasta Carbonara with Zoodles

Zoodles are more than an "alternative" to standard pasta-they're a culinary treat!

With all the smooth textures and the Italian classic's crunchy bacon.

Ingredients

- 1¼ cups heavy whipping cream
- 1 tbsp. butter
- 10 oz. bacon or pancetta, diced
- salt and pepper
- 2 lbs. zucchini - 4 egg yolks
- 3 oz. grated parmesan cheese, for serving

INSTRUCTIONS

Zoodles

Using a spiraling agent to build zoodles. When you do not have a spiral, you can instead use a potato peeler to make zoodles slightly wider.

Bacon

Melt butter over medium heat in a large frying pan. Remove bacon and fry until smooth.

Set the bacon, including the fat, aside and allow to cool.

Sauce

In a medium-high sun, pour heavy cream into a cup and bring to a boil. Stir in a tablespoon of salt. Reduce heat and proceed to boil until the cream is about a quarter down slowly.

Remove the saucepan from heat and raising the temperature of the milk, remove it often to prevent the skin from developing.

Combine the egg yolks, cooked diced bacon with the fat and parmesan cheese in a separate bowl (while the cream is reduced).

Attach the egg-bacon-parmesan blend to a warm sauce and mix continuously to make sure that the egg blend doesn't scramble.

To taste, apply salt and pepper. Return the cup to medium-low heat to steam the sauce softly. Attach the zoodles to the bowl and steam (1-2 minutes).

To serve

Divide into portions and plate of carbonara. Top with an abundance of newly rubbed parmesan

THURSDAY

BREAKFAST

Dairy-free keto latte

Latte? Latte? Yes, please! Yes, please! This milk-free treat is the ideal breakfast on site. Mix it up for 5 minutes and you're done.

Ingredients

- 2 eggs - 2 tbsp. coconut oil
- 1½ cups boiling water
- 1 pinch vanilla extract
- 1 tsp. pumpkin pie spice or ground ginger

INSTRUCTIONS

In a mixer, combine all ingredients. You must be quick so that the eggs do not cook in the boiling water! Drink right away.

TIP! TIP!

Whether you like hot chocolate or even a simple latte, substitute the spices for 1 tablespoon of cocoa or immediate coffee. That's it!

LUNCH

Keto avocado, bacon and goat-cheese salad

Creamy avocados and goat cheese cracked in the nuts? Oh, god. Oh, god. Have we got a recipe for you! Pull it together for a fast lunch or dinner lightening.

INGREDIENTS

- 8 oz. goat cheese
- 8 oz. bacon
- 2 avocados
- 4 oz. arugula lettuce
- 4 oz. walnuts

DRESSING

- 1 tbsp. lemons, the juice
- ½ cup mayonnaise
- ½ cup olive oil
- 2 tbsp. heavy whipping cream
- salt and pepper

INSTRUCTIONS

Preheat the oven to 200 ° F and bring parchment paper into a bakery.

Cut the goat's cheese in half inches round (~1 cm) and placed in the bakery. Bake until golden on the top rack.

In a saucepan, cook the bacon until it is crispy.

Cut the avocado into pieces and put it on top. Attach the bacon and goat cheese to the fried bacon. Sprinkle on top of the nuts. Create the dressing with lemon juice, mayonnaise, olive oil and cream with an immersion blender. Season to taste with salt and pepper.

Tip! Tip!

You're looking for a bit more diversity? While this dressing is all-round, please add your favorite herbs to make it even more irresistible. New parsley, dill or thyme will remarkably well finish off the dressing.

DINNER

Keto pizza

Pizza, eat keto, eat keto. It's a convenient way to fix your pizza without the carbs. Whether it's a simple pepperoni, cheese and tomato sauce, or a charged extravaganza, it's all you want.

Ingredients

- Crust
- 4 eggs
- 6 oz. shredded cheese, preferably mozzarella or provolone
- Topping
- 3 tbsp. unsweetened tomato sauce
- 1 tsp. dried oregano
- 5 oz. shredded cheese
- 1½ oz. pepperoni
- olives (optional)
- For serving
- 2 oz. leafy greens
- 4 tbsp. olive oil
- sea salt and ground black pepper

INSTRUCTIONS

Preheat oven to 200 ° C (400 ° F). Preheat.

Start with the crust. Crack eggs and add shredded cheese to a medium sized cup. Give it a strong mix stir.

Using a spatula on a baking sheet lined with parchment paper to spread the forage and egg batter. You can make two circles or just one big rectangular pizza. Bake for 15 minutes in the oven until the crust is golden. Remove and let it cool for one or two minutes.

Increase temperature of the oven to 225 ° C (450 ° F).

Sprinkle tomato sauce on top and sprinkle with oregano. Place the pepperoni and olives on top of the cheese.

Bake for 5-10 minutes or until the pizza is golden brown.

Serve on the side with a new salad.

FRIDAY

BREAKFAST

Keto mushroom omelet

You are looking for a quick and easy way to start your day? It takes a few minutes to make this hearty omelet super healthy! New champignons make a wonderful filling.

Ingredients

- 3 eggs
- 1 oz. butter, for frying
- 1 oz. shredded cheese
- ¼ yellow onion, chopped
- 4 large mushrooms, sliced
- salt and pepper

INSTRUCTIONS

Crush the eggs in a salt and pepper mixing dish. Whisk the eggs easily and frothily with a brush.

In a frying pan, melt the butter over medium heat. Add the mushrooms and onion to the pan, stir tenderly, then pour into the egg mixture around the vegetables.

When the omelet starts to cook, but still has a little raw egg, sprinkle over the egg. Using a spatula, relieve the omelet carefully and fold it in half. When the golden-brown underneath begins to transform, remove the pot from the heat and push the omelet to a plate.

LUNCH

Keto smoked salmon plate

Ingredients

- ¾ lb. smoked salmon
- 1 cup mayonnaise
- 2 oz. baby spinach
- 1 tbsp. olive oil
- ½ lime (optional)
- salt and pepper

INSTRUCTIONS

Place salmon, spinach, a lime wedge and a hearty mayonnaise doll on a platter.

Drizzle olive oil with salt and pepper over the spinach.

Tip! Tip!

Swap salmon for any fatty fish you want. (Mackerel, herring, sardines and anchovies are all great options.) Greens may also vary — shrimp or spicy arugula.

DINNER

Keto tortilla with ground beef and salsa

Treat yourself to a lovely tortilla filled with meat and cheese. This Mexican favorite will not only be good, but also delicious with your own homemade keto bread and spice blend!

Ingredients

- Low-carb tortillas
- 2 eggs
- 2 egg whites
- 5 oz. cream cheese, softened
- ½ tsp. salt
- 1½ tsp. ground psyllium husk powder
- 1 tbsp. coconut flour

Filling

- 2 tbsp. olive oil
- 1 lb. ground beef or ground lamb, at room temperature
- 2 tbsp. Tex-Mex seasoning
- ½ cup water
- salt and pepper

- Salsa
- 2 avocados, diced
- 1 tomato, diced
- 2 tbsp. lime juice
- 1 tbsp. olive oil
- ½ cup fresh cilantro, chopped
- salt and pepper

For serving
- 6 oz. shredded Mexican cheese
- 3 oz. shredded lettuce

INSTRUCTIONS

Low-carb tortillas

Preheat oven to 200 ° C (400 ° F). Preheat.

Using a whisk-attached electric blender, whisk the eggs and egg whites in soft, ideally for a few minutes. Beat the cream cheese smoothly in a separate big tub. Add the eggs to milk and whisk to a smooth batter with the eggs and cream cheese.

In a small bowl, add salt, psyllium husk and coconut flour. Add the meal mixture to the batter one spoon at a time and start to whisk. Let the batter sit for a couple of minutes, or until it is as thick as an American batter. How easily a batter swells depends on the psyllium husk brand – a trial and error may be required.

Place the parchment paper on each of two baking sheets. Spread the batter thinly (1/4-inch-thick) with a spatula into 4-6 circles or 2 rectangles.

Cook on the top rack for about 5 minutes or more until a little brown turn around the edges of the tortilla. Check the bottom side carefully so that it doesn't flame.

Filling

Place on medium high heat a large frying pan and heat up the oil. Attach the beef to the ground and fry until cooked. Attach the seasoning of tex-mex and water and blend. Cook until most of the water is gone. Taste to see if additional seasoning is required.

Salsa and serving

Create avocado salsa, tomatoes, lime juice, olive oil and new coriander. To taste salt and pepper.

Serve in a tortilla beef filled with shredded cheese, salsa and chopped leafy greens.

Tip! Tip!

Pull the ground beef from the fridge a while before frying. Cold ground beef should cool down the pan and boil and not cook the ground beef. Last tastes even better.

SATURDAY

BREAKFAST

Keto baked bacon omelet

For breakfast, lunch or dinner, bacon. The spinach adds color and color. The eggs keep it together. Yet bacon prevails.

Ingredients
- 4 eggs
- 5 oz. bacon cut in cubes
- 3 oz. butter
- 2 oz. fresh spinach
- 1 tbsp. finely chopped fresh chives (optional)
- salt and pepper

INSTRUCTIONS

Preheat oven to 200 ° C (400 ° F). Preheat. Grease a single serve bakery with butter.

In the remaining fat, cook the bacon and spinach. Whisk the eggs until they are sparkling. Mix the spinach and bacon and fry the left fat.

Add some chopped cabbage. Season with salt and pepper to taste.

Into bakery dish(s), add the egg mixture and bread for 20 minutes or until golden brown.

Let cool and serve for a few minutes.

TIP! TIP!

You might want to add some sprinkled cheddar or sprinkle parmesan on top before baking if you love cheese. Another potential yummy addition is sauteed onions.

LUNCH
Keto quesadillas

Cook up this quick and simple ASAP delight. Decadent. Decadent. Cheesy. Cheesy. And keto officially! Delicious and lovely enough to make you feel like a famous chef. Serve them with sour cream, guacamole and salsa as it is or fried.

Ingredients

- Low-carb tortillas
- Two eggs
- Two egg whites
- 6 oz. Cream cheese
- ½ tsp. salt
- 1½ tsp. ground psyllium husk powder
- 1 tbsp. coconut flour

Filling

- 1 tbsp. olive oil or butter, for frying
- 5 oz. Mexican cheese or any hard cheese of your liking
- 1 oz. baby spinach

INSTRUCTIONS

Tortillas

Preheat oven to 200 ° C (400 ° F). Preheat.

Beat eggs and egg whites together with an electric mixer until fluffy. Apply cream cheese and keep beating until the batter is smooth. Combine salt, psyllium husk and coconut meal in a dish. Mix well. Blend well. Drop the meal mixture into the batter. Let the batter sit for a couple of minutes when combined. It should be as dense as a batter pancake. Your psyllium husk powder brand will affect this step — be patient, if it doesn't thicken enough, add some more.

Placed parchment paper on a sheet of the bakery. Using a spatula to stretch the batter to a wide rectangle on the parchment board. You can cook them in a frying pan like pancakes if you want round tortillas.

Bake for around 5–10 minutes on the top rack, until the tortilla turns brown around its edges. Keep your hand on the oven — don't let this delicious creation burn down!

Cut the big tortilla into smaller pieces (6 pieces per sheet of baking).

Quesadillas

Heat oil or butter over medium heat in a small, non-stick skillet.

In the frying, pot put a tortilla and sprinkle with cheese, spinach and some additional cheese. Top again with a tortilla. Fry each quesadilla on each side for about a minute. You'll know when the cheese melts; it's done.

DINNER
Keto Asian cabbage stir-fry

This vibrant keto fry is not only easy to make, but it is also absolutely delicious. This crunchy pleasure may be one of your favourite recipes. Consider doing it this evening

Ingredients

- 1½ lbs. green cabbage
- 4 oz. butter, divided
- 1 tsp. salt
- 1 tsp.Onion powder
- ¼ tsp. ground black pepper
- 1 tbsp. white wine vinegar
- Two garlic cloves, minced
- 1 tsp. chilli flakes
- 1 tbsp. fresh ginger, finely chopped or grated
- 1¼ lbs. ground beef
- Three scallions, chopped in 1/2-inch slices
- 1 tbsp. sesame oil
- Wasabi mayonnaise
- One cup mayonnaise
- ½ tbsp. wasabi paste

INSTRUCTIONS

Using a sharp knife or food processor to cut the meat finely.

Fry the cabbage in half of the butter on medium to high heat in a large frying or wok pan. It takes a while to soften the chicken, but don't let it turn brown.

Add vinegar and seasoning. Stir and cook for a few more minutes. Place the chicken in a tub.

In the same frying pan, melt the rest of the butter. Remove garlic, flakes of chilli and ginger. Selle for a couple of minutes. Add ground and brown meat until the meat has been fully cooked and most juices evaporate. Only lower the heat a little.

Add meat scallions and chicken. Stir until it's all dry. To taste salt and pepper. Drizzle before serving with sesame seed. Mix wasabi mayonnaise together, starting with a little wasabi, and add more until the taste is right. Serve the warm stir-fry with a wasabi mayonnaise dollop.

SUNDAY

BREAKFAST

Keto pancakes with berries and whipped cream

Try these incredible cheese pancakes, and you can never get back to normal cheese pancakes! Our berry topping gives them the perfect flavour and the children love them as well

Ingredients

- Pancakes
- Four eggs
- 7 oz. cottage cheese
- 1 tbsp. ground psyllium husk powder
- 2 oz. butter or coconut oil

Toppings

- 2 oz. fresh raspberries or fresh blueberries or fresh strawberries
- 1 cup heavy whipping cream

INSTRUCTIONS

In a medium-size bowl, add milk, cottage cheese and psyllium husk and blend together. Enable 5-10 minutes to thicken a little. In a non-stick dish, heat up butter or oil. On medium-low oil, fry the pancakes for 3–4 minutes on each side. Don't make them too wide or they're going to be difficult to flip. Fill a separate bowl with cream and whip until soft peaks are formed. Serve the pancakes with your favourite whipped cream and berries. Lunch

Italian keto plate

Real food on a dish. Mates. Prosciutto. Mozzarella. Mozzarella. Olives and onions. Onions.

Ingredients

- 7 oz. fresh mozzarella cheese
- 7 oz. prosciutto, sliced
- Two tomatoes
- 1⁄3 cup olive oil
- Ten green olives
- salt and pepper

INSTRUCTIONS

Placed on platter tomatoes, prosciutto, cheese and olives. Serve with olive oil and season to taste with salt and pepper. Tip! Tip! Swap the prosciutto for another fatty Italian delicacy. Come to mind soppressata, coppa, or speck. What is your favourite? What is your favourite?

DINNER

Pork chops with green beans and garlic butter

Juicy cuts of pork. Crunchy green beans. White beans. Butter of garlic. This is what we're calling a one-skillet wonder.

Ingredients

- Garlic butter
- 5 oz. Butter, at room temperature
- ½ tbsp. garlic powder
- 1 tbsp. dried parsley
- 1 tbsp. lemon juice
- salt and pepper
- Pork chops

- Four pork chops
- 2 oz. butter, for frying
- 1 lb. fresh green beans
- salt and pepper

INSTRUCTIONS

Add butter, garlic, pets and citrus juice. Blend together. Season to taste with salt and pepper. Set aside. Set aside. Create some small cuts in the fat around the chops to hold them flat during frying. Salt and pepper season. Pack. Melt the butter over medium-high heat in a large frying pan. Fill the chops and fry on each side about 5 minutes or until golden brown and thoroughly fried. Take the chops out of the pot and keep warm. Choose the same pot and add the socks. To taste salt and pepper. Cook over medium-high temperature until the beans are vibrant and slightly fluffy, but still somewhat crunchy. Serve pork chops and beans with a molten dollop of garlic butter. Tip! Tip!

Canned or frozen green beans may not be as crunchy, but they still taste fantastic and deliver basic nutrients from your freezer or pantry.

WEEK 2

MONDAY

BREAKFAST

No-bread keto breakfast sandwich

The ultimate in inventiveness is this sandwich. Scrumptious cheese, sizzling ham and eggs are joined together to create a sandwich – without the pasta! Engineering

INGREDIENTS

- 2 tbsp. butter
- Four eggs
- salt and pepper
- 1 oz. smoked deli ham
- 2 oz. cheddar cheese or provolone cheese or Edam cheese, cut in thick slices
- a few drops of tabasco sauce

INSTRUCTIONS

In a large frying pan, add butter and place over medium heat. Add the eggs and fry on both sides easily. To taste salt and pepper. Using a fried egg as the basis for any sandwich. Place each stack with the ham/pastrami / cold cuts and add the cheese. Top off each fried egg stack. Leave the cheese in the pot, if you want it to melt, at low heat.

Sprinkle a couple of drops of Tabasco or Worcestershire sauce and serve as soon as possible.

Tip! Tip!

The Dijon mustard is a good fit for the ham. Moreover, the ham can be replaced with crispy bacon, or the meat can be skipped entirely. This is a fantastic sandwich paired with a green salad or an avocado!

LUNCH

Keto tuna salad with boiled eggs

Within 15 minutes, a keto meal? Yes, please! Yes, please! Creamy tuna salad served on a crisp salad with perfectly cooked eggs and tomatoes to enhance the dish.

Ingredients

- 4 oz. celery stalks
- Two scallions
- 5 oz. tuna in olive oil
- ½ lemon, zest and juice
- ½ cup mayonnaise
- 1 tsp. Dijon mustard
- Four eggs
- 6 oz. Romaine lettuce
- 4 oz. cherry tomatoes
- 2 tbsp. olive oil
- salt and pepper

INSTRUCTIONS

Chop celery and scallions sweetly. Attach the tuna, lemon, mayonnaise and mustard to a medium-sized cup. Mix and season with salt and pepper. Set aside. Set aside.

To a saucepan, add eggs and add water until the eggs are coated. Bring to a boil and cook for five to six minutes (soft-medium), or for eight to ten (hardboiled) minutes.

When finished, growing the eggs in ice-cold water immediately to make it easier to peel. Divide into coils or halves. Place the tuna mix and eggs on a bed of roman salad. Tomatoes and olive oil on top. Add the tomatoes. Season to taste with salt and pepper.

Tip! Tip!

A generous sprinkle of ground cumin, curry or paprika will give the hard-boiled eggs interesting flavours. Don't skip salt and pepper, however!

You can add a traditional, home-made French vinaigrette if you're not a mayonnaise addict. Simply whisk two tablespoons of red- or white-wine vinegar, squeeze a lemon, five extra virgin olive oil tablespoons, two teaspoons of Dijon mustard and salt and pepper to taste. For a new, moist taste, mix this with the tuna-without mayo!

DINNER

Keto hamburger patties with creamy tomato sauce and fried cabbage

A tasty burger doesn't need bun! Good luck, with a rich tomato sauce, and a side of sautéed chicken.

Ingredients

- Hamburger patties
- 1½ lbs. ground beef
- One egg
- 3 oz. crumbled feta cheese
- 1 tsp.Salt
- ¼ tsp. ground black pepper
- 2 oz. fresh parsley, finely chopped
- 1 tbsp. olive oil, for frying
- 2 tbsp. butter, for frying
- Gravy
- ¾ cup heavy whipping cream
- 1 oz. fresh parsley, coarsely chopped
- 2 tbsp. tomato paste or ajvar relish
- salt and pepper
- Fried green cabbage
- 1½ lbs. shredded green cabbage
- 4½ oz. butter
- salt and pepper

INSTRUCTIONS

Hamburger patties and gravy

In a large bowl, add all the ingredients for the hamburgers. Mix it with a wooden spoon or clean your hands. Don't mix over because your patties can be tough. To shape eight oblong patties, use the wet hands.

In a large frying pan, add butter and olive oil. Fry for at least 10 minutes over medium-high heat or until the patties have turned nice. Flip them for even cooking a few times.

In a small tub, whisk the tomato paste and cream together. Fill in this mixture when the patties are nearly finished. Stir and cook for a couple of minutes. To taste salt and pepper.

Sprinkle chopped pink on top before serving before serving.

Butter-fried green cabbage

Using a food processor or a sharp knife to cut the col finely.

In a large frying pan, add butter.

Place the pot over medium-high heat and sauté the chopped chop for at least 15 minutes or until chopped, golden brown on the edges.

Mix periodically and slightly lower the heat to the top. To taste, apply salt and pepper.

TUESDAY
BREAKFAST
Butter coffee

Butter and coffee oil? Very. Very. A couple of sips of this coffee emulsion hot keto piping, and you are able to take on the universe. Fill 'er up! Fill' er up!

Ingredients

- 1 cup hot coffee freshly brewed
- 2 tbsp. unsalted butter
- 1 tbsp. MCT oil or coconut oil

INSTRUCTIONS

In a mixer, add all ingredients. Blend smoothly and smoothly.

Serve immediately. Serve immediately.

Lunch

Keto roast beef and cheddar plate

Real food on a dish. Beef, cheese and avocado roast. Radishes and scallions crunchy.

Ingredients

- 7 oz. deli roast beef
- 5 oz. cheddar cheese
- One avocado
- Six radishes
- One scallion
- ½ cup mayonnaise
- 1 tbsp. Dijon mustard
- 2 oz. lettuce - 2 tbsp. olive oil
- salt and pepper

INSTRUCTIONS

Place on a platter roast beef, cheese, avocado and radishes.

Attach sliced onion, mustard and a small mayonnaise dollop.

Serve with olive oil and lettuce.

TIP! TIP!

Swap some mayo for butter and use butter and salt to try the radishes. Just perfect!

DINNER
Keto fried salmon with broccoli and cheese

In just half an hour, you can make a delicious, fresh and balanced meal! Salmon and broccoli go together beautifully

Ingredients

- 1 lb. broccoli - 3 oz. butter
- salt and pepper
- 5 oz. grated cheddar cheese
- 1½ lbs. salmon
- One lime

INSTRUCTIONS

Preheat the oven to 400 ° F (200 ° C) with broiler temperature, ideally.

Cut broccoli into smaller florets and simmer for a few minutes in slightly salted water. Ensure the broccoli preserves its chewy texture and delicate colour. Drain and discard the boiling water from the broccoli. Allow, uncovered, for one minute or two to evaporate the steam. Place the drained broccoli in a fat bakery. To taste, add butter and pepper.

Sprinkle the cheese and bake it in the oven for 15-20 minutes or until the cheese is golden.

Meanwhile, season the salmon with salt and pepper and fry them in a lot of butter on each side for a few minutes. The lime may be fried or served raw in the same bowl. You can also take this step on an outdoor grill.

TIP! TIP!

Broccoli may be substituted for other vegetables such as the sprouts of Brussels, green beans or asparagus with little or no change in the number of carbs in the dish. If you want to use some other kind of fish, we recommend other fatty fish like trout or mackerel, but white fish can be used if you prefer.

You can use a combination of different cheeses if you do not like cheddar. Half mozzarella and half parmesan are going to be as fine!

WEDNESDAY
BREAKFAST
Keto coconut porridge
This morning, feel like hot cereal? Check this delight to relax, warm-in-the-beauty comfort food.
Ingredients

- One egg, beaten
- 1 tbsp. coconut flour
- One pinch ground psyllium husk powder
- One pinch salt
- 1 oz. butter or coconut oil
- 4 tbsp. coconut cream

INSTRUCTIONS
Combine the milk, coconut flour, psyllium husk powder and salt in a small cup.
Melt the butter and coconut cream over low heat. Slowly whisk in an egg mixture and then blend until a smooth, dense texture is achieved.
Serve with cream or chocolate milk. Top your porridge and enjoy a few fresh or frozen berries!

LUNCH
Keto shrimp and artichoke plate
Real food on a dish. Shrimp. Shrimp. Cookies. Cookies. Spinach, sun-dried tomatoes and artichokes.
Ingredients

- Four eggs
- 10 oz. cooked and peeled shrimp
- 14 oz. canned artichokes
- Six sun-dried tomatoes in oil
- ½ cup mayonnaise
- 1½ oz. baby spinach
- 4 tbsp. olive oil
- salt and pepper

INSTRUCTIONS
Start to cook the eggs. Reduce them carefully and boil for 4-8 minutes, depending on whether soft or hard-boiled. Refrigerate the eggs in ice-cold water for 1-2 minutes, making the shell easier to remove. On a plate, place eggs, shrimp, artichokes, mayonnaise, tomatoes with sun-dried and spinach. Drizzle the spinach with olive oil. Season to taste and serve with salt and pepper.
Tip! Tip!
Pick up your artichoke hearts and sun-dried tomatoes packed with olive oil for the best flavour.

DINNER
Keto chicken casserole
Keto and casseroles go hand in hand, particularly in this irresistible chicken recipe that will make your whole family swoon. The cream sauce is warm, salty and filled with tasty pesto. Your oven will always be proud to back this tasty goodness for you.
Ingredients

- ¾ cup heavy whipping cream or sour cream
- ½ cup cream cheese
- 3 tbsp. green pesto
- ½ lemon, the juice
- salt and pepper
- 1½ oz. butter
- 2 lbs. skinless, boneless chicken thighs, cut into bite-sized pieces
- One leek, finely chopped
- 4 oz. cherry tomatoes halved
- 1 lb. cauliflower, cut into small florets
- 7 oz. shredded cheese

INSTRUCTIONS

Preheat oven to 200 ° C (400 ° F). Preheat. Pair pesto and lemon juice with milk and cream cheese. To taste salt and pepper. Melt the butter in a big pot over medium heat. Remove chicken, salt and pepper and fry until good golden brown colours. Place the chicken in a 9 x 13 cm (23 x 33 cm) grated baked dish and dump into the mixture of the milk. Leek, tomatoes and cauliflower on top of chicken. Sprinkle the cheese on top and bake for at least 30 minutes in the middle of the oven, or to cook the chicken entirely. If you risk burning the casserole before it is done, cover with aluminium foil, reduce the heat and let cook a little longer.

THURSDAY

BREAKFAST

Keto egg muffins

One of the best time-saving breakfasts of all time. Delicious, savoury eggs are cosy, easy to make and great for adults and children on-the-go! Allow time ahead and rejoice in your preparation!

Ingredients

- Two scallions, finely chopped
- 5 oz. chopped air-dried chorizo or salami or cooked bacon
- 12 eggs
- 2 tbsp. red pesto or green pesto
- salt and pepper
- 6 oz. shredded cheese

INSTRUCTIONS

Preheat oven to 175 ° C (350 ° F). Preheat oven.

Fill a non-stick muffin pan, insertable baking bowls or grate a buttered Silicone Muffin container.

Fill the tin with scallions and chorizo. Whisk eggs and pesto, salt and pepper together. Stir in the cheese and stir. Pour the batter on the chorizo and the scallions.

Bake, depending on the muffin tin size, for 15-20 minutes.

LUNCH

Keto cauliflower soup with crispy pancetta

Any time? Any time? No problem. No problem. This soup demonstrates that keto food can be as fast and as simple as it is deeply satisfying. This is a silky, rich soup with salty pancetta snap, cauliflower and nuts.

Ingredients

- 4 cups chicken broth or vegetable stock
- 1 lb. cauliflower
- 1 tbsp. butter, for frying
- 7 oz. cream cheese
- 1 tbsp. Dijon mustard
- 4 oz. butter
- salt and pepper
- 7 oz. pancetta or bacon, diced
- 1 tsp. paprika powder or smoked chilli powder
- 3 oz. pecans

INSTRUCTIONS

Remove the cauliflower and split into smaller blooms. The smaller you cut, the sooner the soup is ready.

Save a handful of fresh chops and cut into tiny 1/4-inch pieces.

Savour the cauliflower (from phase 2) and pancetta or butter bacon until crispy.

Towards the top, add nuts and paprika powder. Set aside the serving mixture.

Boil the cauliflower in the stock until it is tender. Add milk, butter and mustard.

Blend the soup to the desired consistency, using an immersion blender.

The longer you mix, the more delicious the soup.

To taste salt and pepper.

Serve the soup in bowls and incorporate a variety of fried pancetta.

TIP! TIP!

Like variety, want variety? Then swap your favourite blend of nuts and seeds out of the pecans. And if you have low stock, don't worry. Simply substitute with slightly salted water.

DINNER
Keto cheeseburger

Burgers of Cheese ... What could be your casual feast's most beautiful centrepiece? High on taste and enjoyment, but low on effort! And you don't need bread to make them delicious

Ingredients

- Salsa
- Two tomatoes
- Two scallions - One avocado
- 1 tbsp. olive oil
- salt
- fresh cilantro, to taste
- Burgers
- 1½ lbs. ground beef
- 7 oz. shredded cheese, divided
- 2 tsp. garlic powder - 2 tsp. onion powder
- 2 tsp. paprika powder
- 2 tbsp. fresh oregano, finely chopped
- 2 oz. butter, for frying
- Salt & pepper, to taste

Toppings

- 5 oz. lettuce
- ¾ cup mayonnaise
- 5 oz. cooked bacon, crumbled
- 4 tbsp. pickled jalapeños, chopped
- 2½ oz. sliced dill pickles
- 4 tbsp. Dijon mustard

INSTRUCTIONS

Cut the salsa ingredients in a small bowl and mix together. Set aside. Set aside.

In seasoning, mix with half the cheese into ground beef and blend with the hands or a wooden spoon.

Create four burgers and fry if you want in a pan or grill.

Cover with salt and pepper and add the rest of the cheese on top.

Serve on mayo salad, bacon, jalapeño pickled, dill pickle and mustard. And don't forget the salsa home-made!

Tip! Tip!

This is how you can make your own super safe mayonnaise free of soybean oil and additives

FRIDAY
BREAKFAST
Boiled eggs with mayonnaise

Egg lovers, gather around! Gather around! This recipe is so simple, so delicious and just what your body needs to feel happy.

Ingredients

- Eight eggs
- 8 tbsp. mayonnaise
- Two avocados

INSTRUCTIONS

Bring water in a pot to a boil.

Optional: In the shells, make tiny wholes with an egg piercer. It helps to avoid cracking eggs during boiling.

Place the eggs carefully in the bowl.

For soft-boiled eggs, boil the egg for 5-6 minutes, medium for 6-8 minutes, and hard-boiled eggs for 8-10 minutes.

Serve with mayonnaise. Mayonnaise. Suggestion for service

Enjoy your breakfast with some avocado, or fried mayonnaise asparagus.

One really simple choice is to eat the boiled buttered eggs.

Mash them in a small bowl together.

When you're in the mood, add some new herbs.

Delicious!

Delicious!

Lunch

Keto Caesar salad

A true classic keto salad: Moist chicken and crispy bacon are served in a Roman lettuce spread.

Ingredients

- ¾ lb. chicken breasts
- 1 tbsp. olive oil
- salt and pepper - 3 oz. bacon
- 7 oz. Romaine lettuce
- 1 oz. parmesan cheese, freshly grated
- Dressing - ½ cup mayonnaise
- 1 tbsp. Dijon mustard
- ½ lemon, zest and juice
- ½ oz. grated parmesan cheese, finely grated
- 2 tbsp. finely chopped filets of anchovies
- One garlic clove, pressed or finely chopped
- salt and pepper

Instructions

Preheat oven to 175 ° C (350 ° F). Preheat oven.

Mix the dressing ingredients with a whisk or dip blender. Set aside in the fridge.

In a greased baking dish, put the chicken breasts.

Apply salt and pepper to the chicken and rice olive oil or melted butter over the top. Bake the chicken for about 20 minutes in the oven or until fully cooked. The chicken can also be cooked on the stovetop if you prefer.

Fry the bacon to smooth. Cut the lettuce and put on two plates as a base. Place the crispy, crumbled bacon and the chicken on top.

Finish with a generous dressing doll and a nice grill of parmesan cheese.

Dinner

Fathead pizza

Mouthwatering. Mouthwatering. Satisfactory. All your favourite aromas of pizza layered over a crunchy, cheesy, keto crust. Great ever pizza

Ingredients

- Topping
- 8 oz. fresh Italian sausage
- 1 tbsp.Butter
- ½ cup unsweetened tomato sauce
- ½ tsp. dried oregano
- 5 oz. mozzarella cheese, shredded
- Crust
- 6 oz. mozzarella cheese, shredded
- 2 tbsp. cream cheese
- ¾ cup almond flour
- 1 tsp. white wine vinegar
- One egg - ½ tsp. salt
- olive oil, to grease your hands

Instructions

Preheat oven to 200 ° C (400 ° F). Preheat.

In a medium-heat non-stick pot, heat mozzarella and cream cheese, or in a pan in a microwave oven. Remove until they're melting together. Add the remaining ingredients and combine well. Tip: use a dough hook hand blender. Humidify your hands and flatten the dough with olive oil on parchment paper, making a circle around 8 "(20 cm) in diameter. A rolling pin can also be used to flatten the dough between two sheets of parchment paper.

Remove the top sheet of parchment (if used). Pinch the crust with a dip (all over) and bake for 10-15 minutes in the oven until the brown is golden. Remove from oven. Detach from the oven.

Drizzle the ground sausage meat in olive oil or butter while the crust is baking.

Spread on the crust a thin layer of tomato sauce. Place meat and plenty of cheese on top of the pizza. Bake until cheese has melted for 10–15 minutes. Sprinkle oregano with it and enjoy it!

SATURDAY
BREAKFAST
Classic bacon and eggs

Some of the best breakfasts in the world! Take this mouthwatering version to your bacon and egg game. Measure your hunger meter and enjoy as many eggs as you like.

Ingredients

- Eight eggs
- 5 oz. bacon, in slices
- cherry tomatoes
- fresh parsley

INSTRUCTIONS

In a medium heat dish, fry the bacon until crispy. Placed on a plate aside. Leave the fat in the pot.

Use the same pot to sprinkle the eggs. Crack your eggs into the bacon grate over medium heat. You may also break them into a measuring cup and bring them into the pan carefully so that the heat is not splattered. Cook the eggs whatever you like. To the sunny side — fry the eggs on one side and cover with a sheet to make sure they are fried. For eggs that are quickly cooked, turn the eggs after a few minutes and cook again. Break the cherry tomatoes in half and immediately fry them.

To taste salt and pepper.

LUNCH
Keto salmon-filled avocados

Avocado + salmon smoked = no cooking. This creamy dish is a delicious breakfast, quick lunch or light dinner.

Ingredients

- Two avocados
- 6 oz. smoked salmon
- ¾ cup crème Fraiche or sour cream or mayonnaise
- salt and pepper
- 2 tbsp. lemon juice

INSTRUCTIONS

Halve the avocados and remove the hole.

In the hollow of the avocado, put a dollop of crème Fraiche or mayonnaise and add the smoked salmon over it.

Check salt and a squeeze of lemon juice for extra flavour (and prevent the avocado from turning brown).

Tip! Tip!

Any other form of fatty fish — boiled, fried or smoked — can be eaten on this keto.

With a little fresh dill, it tastes even better!

DINNER
Keto ribeye steak with oven-roasted vegetables

Let's get down to the matter's red meat.

In this scenario, a perfectly cured rivet steak with anchovy butter.

And so, so, it's easy to construct.

Ingredients

- 1 lb. broccoli
- One whole garlic
- 10 oz. cherry tomatoes
- 3 tbsp. olive oil
- 1 tbsp. dried thyme or dried oregano or dried basil
- 1½ lbs.rib-eye steaks
- salt and pepper
- Anchovy butter
- 1 oz. anchovies
- 5 oz. butter, at room temperature
- 1 tbsp. lemon juice
- salt and pepper

INSTRUCTIONS

Create the butter of anchovy. Chop the anchovy fillets finely and blend with butter (at room temperature), lemon juice, salt and pepper. Set aside. Set aside. Preheat your oven to 450 ° F (225 ° C) and make sure that your meat is out of the fridge before cooking. Separate the cloves from the garlic, but do not peel them. Cut broccoli into bloom. You can include them in the stem, only peel off any raw pieces and slice them.

Grease a large roasting pot and put in a single layer all the vegetables. Top with olive oil season and drizzle. Place the roasting pot in the oven for 15 minutes. Swirl to cover.

Clean the meat with olive oil and salt and pepper. Fry easily in a frying pan on high heat. You just want to give the meat a good seated surface at this stage. Remove the pot from the oven and place between the vegetables for the meat.

Lower the heat to 400 ° F (200 ° C) and bring a few minutes back into the oven to 10 or 15, depending on whether your meat is fine-fresh, medium or well-done. Remove from the oven and every on every piece of meat a dollop of anchovy butter. Serve immediately.

Tip! Tip!

This dish can be made with pork shoulder, chicken or shrimp. Adjust the oven time accordingly. We recommend trying out our other flavoured butter for more variety.

SUNDAY

BREAKFAST

Keto western omelette

Fluffy, cheesy, egg flavour – this is even better than what you serve in the dining room! It is the perfect recipe, burst with delicious bacon, peppers and onions.

Ingredients

- Six eggs
- 2 tbsp. heavy whipping cream or sour cream
- salt and pepper - 3 oz. shredded cheese, divided
- 2 oz. butter
- 5 oz. smoked deli ham, diced
- ½ yellow onion, finely chopped
- ½ green bell pepper, finely chopped

INSTRUCTIONS

Whisk eggs and cream in a mixing bowl until fluffy. Remove salt and potatoes.

Attach half the cheese shredded and blend well.

In a large frying pan, melt the butter over medium heat.

For a few minutes, sauté the diced ham, onion and peppers. Attach the egg blend and fry until almost firmly omelette. Be careful not to burn the edges.

After a while, raising the heat. Sprinkle on top the remainder of the milk. If necessary, fold the omelette.

Serve right away ... And relax! And love!

LUNCH

Keto prosciutto-wrapped asparagus with goat cheese

The complete trio of flavours is rendered by crisp and succulent asparagus, smooth goat cheese and salty prosciutto. So nice, if you would have dressed up, you'll wonder. You're not going to think about it, so easy. And you'll make it so quick every night of the week

Ingredients

- 12 pieces of green asparagus
- 2 oz. prosciutto, in thin slices
- 5 oz. Goat cheese - ¼ tsp. ground black pepper
- 2 tbsp. olive oil

INSTRUCTIONS

Preheat your oven to 450 ° F (225 ° C), with the broiler feature preferably.

Wash the asparagus and cut it.

Cut the cheese into 12 pieces, then split every slice into two pieces.

Cut the slices of prosciutto lengthwise in two sections, and wrap them around one asparagus and two cheese sections.

Located in a bakery filled with parchment paper. Add pepper and olive oil to drizzle.

Cook about 15 minutes in the oven until golden brown.

DINNER
Creamy keto fish casserole
Whitefish swimming in a rich and creamy casserole gets a hint of capper bite and broccoli and greens freshness in it.
Ingredients

- 2 tbsp. olive oil
- 1 lb. broccoli
- Six scallions
- 2 tbsp. small capers
- 1 oz. butter, for greasing the casserole dish
- 1½ lbs. white fish, in serving-sized pieces
- 1¼ cups heavy whipping cream
- 1 tbsp. Dijon mustard
- 1 tsp.Salt
- ¼ tsp. ground black pepper
- 1 tbsp. dried parsley
- 3 oz. butter
- For serving
- 5 oz. leafy greens

INSTRUCTIONS
Preheat oven to 200 ° C (400 ° F). Preheat.

Divide broccoli, including the stem, into tiny blooms. Peel if the stem is tough with a sharp knife or a potato peeler.

Freeze broccoli in medium-high oil for five minutes, until golden and smooth. Salt and pepper season. Pack.

Add scallions, chopped finely, and capers. Fry 1-2 minutes more and bring the vegetables into a grated pastry. Nestle the fish between the vegetables.

Mix parsley, cream and mustard together. Place the fish and vegetables over them. Cover with butter slices.

Bake for 20 minutes or until the fish is cooked and blast with a fork quickly. Serve as it is or with a green salad.

Tip! Tip!

Switch little things up! Salmon and tuna (fresh or frozen) make excellent white fish replacements. And, if broccoli-haters come to dinner, sprinkle, asparagus and mushrooms in Brussels. Using your imagination and never get boring this all-in-one meal.

WEEK 3

MONDAY
BREAKFAST
Portobello egg & avocado "toasts."
Ingredients

- Four portobello mushrooms
- ⅓ cup olive oil
- One tomato
- 1 ½ tbsp. minced garlic
- Four eggs
- One avocado
- 1 tbsp. thyme

INSTRUCTION
Wipe the portobello cap with a damp towel or paper. Heat 2 tbsp.Olive oil in a medium-high heat pot until they shimmer.

In the skillet, place portobello, gills side up and cook until browned, approximately 5 minutes. Flip and cook for another four minutes on the other side. Retire from the pot and put the gill side on a plate. Season to taste with salt and pepper.

Add 2 tbsp.More olive oil to the pot and return to medium to high heat. Cut thick (1-inch) tomato pieces and put them in the pot, cook for a little, and 2 to 3 minutes on each side. Lift from the bowl and stack the top of the pot.

Add the other 2 tbsp.Olive oil and add garlic, then crack an egg(s) on top and fry to taste, 2-3 minutes per hand. Season to taste with salt and pepper.

Slice the avocado thinly and stack on top of the tomato. Place an egg on top of the stack and decorate with new thyme leaves.

LUNCH
Pesto chicken zucchini noodles
Ingredients

- Four zucchinis
- 12 oz. chicken breast, sliced into strips
- 1 ½ tbsp. butter
- ½ cup chicken broth
- ½ cup cream
- ½ cup pesto
- 1 cup shredded parmesan cheese

INSTRUCTION

Peel the turquoise lengthwise into long, thin strips using a vegetable peeler. (Otherwise, use a loop or a sharp knife.) Stick with a paper towel and set aside.

Season with salt and pepper chicken. Heat butter over medium heat in a bowl. Attach the chicken and cook,occasionally stirring, for 8 minutes until fully cooked. Move to board. Switch to board.

Add chicken broth over medium heat to the empty skillet and brush all browned bits off the bottom of the bowl. Reduce the liquid by half to medium-low, then add milk, pesto and 1⁄2 cup parmesan cheese. Simmer and stir periodically, until warmed up for 3 minutes.

Stir in the skillet the chicken and the zucchini noodles; stir in the sauce. Cook for 5 minutes until courgettes have softened and the chicken is cooked. Season to taste with salt and pepper.

Divide into bowls and top with 1⁄2 cup parmesan remaining.

DINNER
Asparagus, bacon and egg bake
Ingredients

- Eight bacon strips
- 8 oz. asparagus
- Eight eggs
- 1 cup shredded mozzarella cheese

Steps

Preheat the oven to 425 ° F. Grease the bakery platter.

Place bacon over medium heat in a large skillet. Cook, regularly roll until fully fried, but not crispy. Switch to a board lined with towels of paper.

During cooking, snap the hard ends of the asparagus off. When bacon is finished, remove the pot from the heat and add the rendered fat to the empty bowl. Cook and powder with salt and pepper. Switch asparagus to the bakery and bake for eight minutes, or until slightly softened. Take from the oven the baking dish and add bacon. Crack the eggs over the top and scatter with mozzarella shredded. Turn back to the oven and bake for five to eight minutes or until your favourite eggs are cooked.

TUESDAY
BREAKFAST
Keto Pancakes
Ingredients

- Almond Flour Pancakes
- 50 grams of Almond Flour
- 50 grams Heavy Whipping Cream
- 1 Egg
- 1 Tbsp. Maple Flavored Syrup
- 1/2 Tsp. Vanilla Extract
- 1/2 Tsp. Baking Powder
- Lily's Chocolate Chips
- a pinch of salt

Coconut Flour Pancakes

- 15 grams Coconut Flour
- 30 grams Heavy Whipping Cream
- 1 Egg
- 1 Tbsp. Maple Flavored Syrup

- 1/2 Tsp. Baking Powder
- 1/2 Tsp. Vanilla Extract
- a pinch of salt
- Chocolate Chips

INSTRUCTIONS

The way all pancakes are made is pretty much the same. In a pot, combine all the ingredients. If you may, I would encourage you to sift your cocoa flour and even almond flour. Then bring all the dry ingredients first into the bowl and then into the wet ones, or first add the wet ones, then add a decent mixture and then combine the dry ones. Any way is perfect, really.

Cook the pancakes in a frying pan in some butter or olive oil/avocado oil. When the butter is melted into a batter ladle, keep the heat low/medium. After the batter is poured, sprinkle the chocolate chips and cover and cook for about two minutes with the lid, and then turn over and cook for another 30 to 45 seconds.

You should combine the chocolate chips with the batter, but I chose to add them later in my own experiments. It's your option either way. Cook all the pancakes and eat them with butter and Keto syrup. Love! Love!

LUNCH

Bell pepper "nachos" with ground beef & cheddar

Ingredients

- ¾ tsp.Chilli powder
- ¼ tsp.Cumin
- ¼ tsp.Garlic powder
- ¼ tsp.Dried oregano
- ¼ tsp. red pepper flakes
- 4 oz. ground beef
- 4 oz. sliced bell peppers
- ½ cup shredded cheddar cheese
- ½ tomato
- ½ avocado
- 2 tbsp. sour cream
- ¼ jalapeno pepper

Steps

Combine chilli powder, cumin, garlic powder, dried oregano, red pepper packets, salt and pepper in a small cup.

In a pot over medium heat, brown ground beef can break up all clumps with the back of a wooden spoon, until it is cooked for around 7 to 10 minutes. Remove the spice mixture and blend properly. Remove from fire. Remove from heat.

Preheat 400 degrees F in the oven. Bring together a sheet of baking paper or aluminium foil. Within a single plate, place bell peppers, close together.

Sprinkle the mixture of ground beef and cheddar over peppers to cover evenly. Bake for 6 to 8 minutes until cheese is melted and bubbly.

For the meantime, tell tomato. Avocado peel and dice.

Top with tomato and avocado peppers and savoury cream and jalapeno (if used). Divide and enjoy on bowls!

DINNER

Red pepper & fontina cauliflower pizza

Ingredients

- 4 cups cauliflower
- One egg
- ½ cup shredded parmesan cheese
- ½ tsp. salt
- ¼ tsp. garlic powder
- ¼ cup almond flour
- 8 oz. fontina
- ¾ cup roasted red peppers
- ¼ cup olive oil
- ½ cup chopped basil

Steps

Preheat the oven to 425 ° F. Line a parchment paper sheet plate.

Shave the cauliflower with a box grater or food processor to a rice-like consistency. Put on high 3 minutes in a large microwave-safe bowl and microwave. Stir and microwave for another 2 minutes. Put aside for coolness.

Squeeze out cauliflower liquid and return to the pot. Remove milk, parmesan, butter, powdered garlic and almond meal. Combine well with your face.

Move the mixture to the ready breadboard and press into a disk, roughly 1/2 inch thick. Cook or golden for 12 minutes. Cook.

In the meantime, slice the fontina thinly and roast the red peppers.

Clean the olive oil crust and cover it with roasted red peppers and fontina. Placed in the oven for three minutes before the cheese starts to melt. Remove with basil from the oven and roof. Cut into bits and have fun!

WEDNESDAY

BREAKFAST

Breakfast Sausage

The best Keto breakfast is a delicious spicy pork sausage

Ingredients

- 250 grams Ground Pork
- 1/2 Tsp. Fennel Seeds
- 1/2 Tsp. Whole Black Peppercorns
- 1/2 Tsp. Sea Salt
- 1/4 Tsp. White Pepper
- 1/4 Tsp. Garlic Powder
- 1/4 Tsp. Smoked Paprika
- 1/8 Tsp. Nutmeg Powder
- 1 Tbsp. Olive Oil/Bacon Fat/Butter/Ghee for frying

INSTRUCTIONS

Grind the sea salt, pepper grains and fennel to produce a spice blend in a mortar and pestle.

Add a tablespoon or so from the freshly ground spice mix along with paprika, white pepper, garlic powder and nutmeg powder to a large mixing bowl. Give it to a good mix and then shape the sausage like a patty using a ring mould or cookie cutter. I recommend 50 grams of meat per slice of sausage. Depending on your choice, you can make them bigger or smaller.

Heat the cooking fat in an iron cast pot or fry pan, then fry the sausage for around 3-4 minutes on either side.

LUNCH

Sausage and green beans with garlic butter

Ingredients

- 1 lb. green beans
- One lemon
- 1 lb. pork sausage
- ⅓ cup butter
- 2 ½ tbsp.Minced garlic
- ¾ tsp. red pepper flakes
- One ¾ tsp.Italian seasoning
- 1 tbsp. thyme
- ½ cup chicken broth

Steps

For microwave health, arrange green beans; add 2 cups of lemon juice and 1 cup of water. Cover and microwave for six minutes, but still tightly steamed. Hold protected and reserve.

Place pork sausage in a skillet for medium heat while green beans are cooking. Attach 2 cups of water, partly cover, cook for 10 minutes and sometimes switch sausages.

When the pot is drained, add 2 tbsp.Butter, 4 tsp.Garlic and red pepper flakes. Cook 2 to 3 minutes uncovered until sausages are slightly browned. Move the sausage to a dish and hold.

Return skillet to medium-low heat, then adds 4 tbsp.Butter, 4 tsp.Garlic, Italian seasoning, thyme, and green beans. Cook, frequently stirring, around four minutes until green beans are well coated in butter and tender.

Add chicken broth to the pot and let thicken for 2 to 3 minutes. Return sausages to the pan and cook about 2 minutes until hot. Shortly before serving, squeeze extra lemon juice on green beans.

DINNER
Prosciutto-wrapped chicken with mushroom sauce
The simple chicken dinner comes with crispy prosciutto and rich champagne sauce.
Ingredients
- Four small chicken breast fillets
- Two spring onions, finely chopped
- 150g Primo Gourmet Selection Prosciutto
- 20g butter
- 200g small Swiss brown mushrooms, thickly sliced
- Two cloves garlic, crushed
- Two tablespoons dry sherry
- 300ml cooking cream
- One tablespoon Dijon mustard
- Two teaspoons honey
- Sliced roast Brussels sprouts, to serve, optional

METHOD
Preheat oven to fan-forced 180C/160C. Line a non-stick baking paper oven plate. Season with pepper per chicken breast. Disseminate the spring onions on top of each fillet. Wrap in prosciutto and put in a ready tray. Bake 35-40 minutes or until the prosciutto is slightly crooked and chicken is cooked. Book tray juices.
In a big, non-stick bowl, melt butter over medium-low heat. Stir in the mushrooms and cook for 4-5 minutes, or until golden brown smooth. If the mushrooms need moisture, add a splash of water. Stir in garlic and cook 1 minute. Shake and cook for 1 minute. Shake. Mix together cream, mustard and sweetheart. Cook sauce for 1-2 minutes until thickened slightly. Add reserved pan juices and season thoroughly and cook 1 minute later. Remove from fire. Remove from heat. Break the chicken into thick bits or leave the plate whole. Swallow on the sauce and serve Brussels sprouts with crispy roasted.

THURSDAY
BREAKFAST
Keto Omurice
Ingredients
- 200 grams Cauliflower Riced
- 180 grams Boneless Chicken Leg and Thigh Meat
- 100 grams White Mushrooms
- 100 grams Tomato Puree
- 30 grams Spring Onion
- 10 grams garlic
- 30 ml Heavy Cream
- 1 Tbsp. olive oil
- 1 Tbsp. Butter
- 1 Tbsp. Rice Wine Vinegar
- 1 Tbsp. Soya Sauce
- 4 Eggs
- 1 Tsp. olive oil For frying the egg
- 1 Tsp. Butter For Frying the egg
- Coriander or Spring Onion Greens For garnish
- Salt & Pepper
- Stevia or preferred sweetener to taste

INSTRUCTIONS
Begin by cutting the mushrooms and onion in the spring. Cut the chicken into bite pieces and purée the tomato if you use a fresh one.
Use the grater attachment of your food processor to rice the cauliflower. Add salt and microwave for 5 minutes and then mix well.
In a frying pan, heat 1 tbsp.Of olive oil and 1 tbsp.Of butter.
Add onions and cook for a minute in the spring. Then apply salt and pepper to the chicken and season.
Add the champagne and sautee to high heat.
Once the mushrooms are released, add the tomato purée, minced garlic, vinegar, soy sauce and stevia sweetener.

Cook until the sauce is a good thick syrup, and add to the cooked colic rice.

Give all this a decent mix and cook for a minute or two and garnish with greens of spring onion or fresh coriander.

Crack two eggs in a mug, add a heavy cream tablespoon and whisk together.

Heat in your oven a tsp. of olive oil and butter

Pour the eggs in and scratch them with chopsticks and continue to move the pot. Once an omelette is made, add half the fried rice of the cauliflower and fold the omelette. Echo the second cycle

Serve with hot sauce or simply eat it as it is.

LUNCH
Keto satay chicken
After the ketogenic diet, favourites to take are not limited. Only skip the rice and select zoodles to make this satay comfortable.
Ingredients

- 1 1/2 tablespoons peanut oil
- Two garlic cloves, crushed
- One teaspoon curry powder
- One teaspoon finely grated fresh ginger
- 2 (125g each) chicken thigh fillets
- 1/4 red onion, finely chopped
- 1/2 small fresh red chilli, deseeded, finely chopped
- One tablespoon peanut butter
- 80ml (1/3 cup) coconut milk
- One teaspoon soy sauce
- 1 1/2 tablespoons chopped roasted salted peanuts
- 1/4 lime, juiced
- One large zucchini, trimmed
- 1/2 Lebanese cucumber, thinly sliced
- 125g cherry tomatoes halved

METHOD

Combine in a low glass or ceramic dish one cubicle of oil, one garlic clove, 1/2 teaspoon of curry powder and ginger. Add the chicken to the coat and turn. Cover and marinate in the refrigerator for at least one hour.

Heat the remaining oil over medium heat in a small cup. Cook the onion, stirring or softening for 3 minutes. Stir the chilli and the rest of the garlic, add the curry powder and cook for 1 minute or until aromatic. Mix the peanut butter, coconut milk and soy sauce together. Simmer, stir, for 2-3 minutes or until slightly thickened. Book 1 teaspoon of peanuts chopped for serving. Remove the rest of the peanuts and lime juice into the sauce. Setback, filled with water.

In between, use a spiralizer to cut the courgettes into long noodles or to cut the courgettes into long streaks with a vegetable peeler. Heat a medium-high heat grill or grill. Cook the chicken on each side for 3-4 minutes or until it is slightly cooked. Transfer to a plate and set aside for 5 minutes before slicing thickly.

Divide the 'noodles' of the courgettes into bowls. Then sprinkle the rice, cucumber and tomatoes with a mild satay sauce.

DINNER
Keto Swedish meatballs
These fast Swedish meatballs make a weekend dream dinner
Ingredients

- 500g beef mince
- One egg
- Four green shallots, thinly sliced
- 1/4 cup finely chopped fresh continental parsley
- One garlic clove, crushed
- One teaspoon allspice
- 1/4 teaspoon ground nutmeg
- Two tablespoons extra virgin olive oil
- 80ml (1/3 cup) Massel Beef Style Liquid Stock
- Two teaspoons Dijon mustard
- 180ml (3/4 cup) pouring cream
- 600g steamed cauliflower, coarsely chopped

- 150g fresh green beans, steamed
- Fresh continental parsley leaves, coarsely chopped, to serve

METHOD

In a big bowl put together beef, potato, shallot, pepper, garlic, allspice and nutmeg. Season well. Season well. Form tablespoonful's into balls of the mixture.

Heat the oil over medium-high heat in a large non-stick frying dish. Cook meatballs, regularly turn, 6-8 minutes, or only cook golden. Move to board. Switch to board.

Into the bowl, add mouth and 125ml (1/2 cup) cream and bring to a boil. Reduce heat and cook for 5 minutes or until halved. Place the meatballs back into the pot and cook for 1-2 minutes or until hot.

In a food processor, position the cauliflower and remaining cream and process until smooth. Saison. Saison.

Divide the chocolate mash between serving plates. Cover the rice, balls of meat and sauce. Saison. Saison. Serve with parsley scattered.

FRIDAY

BREAKFAST

Lemon & Poppy Seed Muffins

A delicious, pleasant Keto muffin, a dessert, breakfast or snack.

Ingredients

- 140 grams of Almond Flour
- 85 grams Butter
- 85 grams Sour Cream
- 100 grams Sukrin Gold (or low carb sweetener of choice)
- 23 grams Poppy Seeds
- 1/2 Tsp. Vanilla Extract
- 1/2 Tsp. Baking Powder
- 2 Eggs
- Juice of a lemon
- the zest of 1 lemon
- a pinch of sea salt

INSTRUCTIONS

In a cup, blend the almond flour, poppy seeds, bakery powder, salt and the citrus fruit and combine with a fork.

For another tub, the butter and the sweetener together. Do not use a granulated sweetener (except if you do not use Keto and sugar), because then they would be hard to remove and safer to be able to powder them.

Then apply the sour cream to the mixture of butter and sweetener and whisk together.

Then add cinnamon, lemon juice and eggs and whisk together. If the mixture appears a little curdled or broken, don't be worried, this is normal. Then add to the wet and whisk dry ingredients until you have a good smooth batter.

Put the batter on cupcake/muffin liners and bake at 175C for approximately 25-30 minutes. Don't forget your oven preheat.

Let them cool at least 20 minutes before digging in until ready.

LUNCH

Easy keto chicken chow mein

INGREDIENTS

- Two tablespoons peanut oil
- 500g chicken thigh fillets, thinly sliced
- 250g broccoli, cut into florets
- Four garlic cloves, thinly sliced
- One long fresh red chilli, deseeded, finely chopped
- extra fresh chilli, finely chopped, to serve
- 1/4 small red cabbage, sliced
- 250g zucchini noodles
- 110g (2 cups) trimmed bean sprouts
- 75g (1/2 cup) roasted unsalted cashew nuts
- Two tablespoons gluten-free soy sauce
- Two teaspoons sesame oil
- Fresh coriander sprigs, to serve

METHOD

Heat half the peanut oil over high heat in a broad wok. Stir-fry for 2-3 minutes half the chicken or golden. Move to board. Switch to board. Undo the rest of the food.

Heat in the wok the rest of the peanut oil. Brush the broccoli, garlic and chilli until soft, crisp, for 2 minutes. Attach the chicken and courgettes. Stir-fry 1 minute, or tenderly.

Switch the chicken back to the wok along with the rice, cassava, and soy and sesame oil. Stir-fry until combined for 1 minute. Serve with coriander, and extra chilli brushed.

DINNER
Tuscan-style chicken
INGREDIENTS

- 1kg chicken pieces on the bone
- One brown onion, thickly sliced
- Two garlic cloves, crushed
- 2 tsp. ground paprika
- 125g semi-dried tomatoes
- 320g jar grilled eggplant, drained, chopped
- 280g jar chargrilled peppers (capsicum), drained, thickly sliced
- 1 cup (160g) pitted mixed olives
- 1/2 cup (125ml) thickened cream
- 1 1/2 cups (375ml) Coles Real Chicken Salt Reduced Stock
- 1/4 cup coarsely chopped oregano

METHOD

Preheat the oven to a temperature of 150 ° C. Place over high heat a big flameproof roasting saucepan. Attach half the chicken, add half the chicken. Cook, turn periodically, 5 minutes or all over until dark. Switch to a heat-resistant mug. Undo the rest of the food.

Stir in the ointment and cook for 5 minutes or until the onion softens. Remove the garlic and paprika, then cook for 1 minute or until flavorful. Tomatoes, eggplant, capsicum, lemon, cream and oregano in the chicken. Bring to a frying pan. Remove from fire. Remove from heat.

Cover and bake for 1 1/4 hours or until chicken are very tender and the sauce slightly thickens. Serving season.

SATURDAY
BREAKFAST
Keto Dosa with Coconut Chutney
A great Indian savoury crepe made of chutney coconut
Ingredients

- For the Dosa
- 18 grams of Almond Flour
- 15 grams Shredded Mozzarella
- 30 ml Coconut Milk
- Salt to Taste
- a pinch Cumin Powder
- a pinch Hing or Asafoetida
- For the Coconut Chutney
- 100 grams of Coconut meat
- 10 grams Ginger
- 1 Green Chilly
- 1 Tbsp. Coconut Oil
- 1 Tsp. Curry Leaves
- 1/2 Tsp. Mustard Seeds
- 1 Dried Red Chilly
- Salt to Taste
- a pinch Hing optional

INSTRUCTIONS

For the Dosa

Combine all the ingredients and make the batter

In a lightly oiled, non-stick, fry and spread batter.

Cook over medium heat until the bottom is brown and the batter cooks all over, and the sides start rising a little off the saucepan.

Fold over the coconut chutney and serve

For the Chutney

Mix the coconut, cool, salt and ginger along with a little water for a coarse chutney.

In a pot heat the coconut oil and add it to the mustard, dried red chilly, curry leaves and hinges.

When the mosquito seeds begin to pop, pour the hot oil and spices over the chutney and mix well.

Eat dosa keto. Eat dosa keto.

LUNCH

Keto creamy chicken and cauliflower salad

INGREDIENTS

- 500g cauliflower, cut into florets
- Two tablespoons olive oil
- One teaspoon Massel chicken style stock powder
- 80ml (1/3 cup) Massel chicken-style stock
- 80ml (1/3 cup) pure cream
- Three teaspoons wholegrain mustard
- One tablespoon chopped fresh chives, plus extra to serve
- Two teaspoons lemon juice
- 400g chicken tenderloins
- 100g streaky bacon
- 100g baby spinach
- 100g rocket leaves
- 60g (1/3 cup) roasted macadamia nuts, chopped

METHOD

Preheat the oven to a forced fan at 200 ° C/180 ° C. Fill a bakery tray with pastry paper. On the prepared tray, place the cauliflower. Sprinkle with 1 1/2 tablespoon oil and stock powder. Bake until golden and tender for 25 minutes.

In the meantime, put stock and mustard in a small bowl and heat to boil. Reduce heat and cook 2 minutes. Remove cream and cook for 2-3 minutes or until sauce is halved. Remove the cabbage and lemon juice and keep dry.

In the large non-stick frying pan, heat remaining oil over medium-high heat. Cook chicken and bacon on each side for three to four minutes, or until golden and crisp. Cut bacon into pieces of 3 cm.

On a serving plate, mix the salad leaves, chicken, cauliflower and bacon. Sprinkle with the cream sauce and sprinkle with the remaining macadamic nuts and cabbage.

DINNER

Keto frappuccino slice

INGREDIENTS

- Two tablespoons boiling water
- 2 1/2 teaspoons gelatine powder
- 250g cream cheese, at room temperature, chopped
- Two tablespoons powdered stevia
- 80ml (1/3 cup) strong espresso coffee, cooled
- One teaspoon vanilla extract
- 300ml thickened cream, whipped, plus extra, whipped, to serve
- Coffee beans, to serve (optional)
- Cacao powder, to dust

BASE

- 100g (1 cup) pecans
- 130g (1 1/4 cups) almond meal
- One tablespoon cacao powder
- One tablespoon powdered stevia

- One egg
- Two tablespoons unsalted butter, melted

METHOD

Preheat oven forced to 180C/160C fan. Cover a 16 x 26 cm slice pot with baking paper to overhang two long sides of the plate. Place the pecans in a food processor and grind them to the ground finely. Apply meal, cacao and stevia to the almond. Combine pulse. Pour in the egg and butter. Actor until the mixture is mixed. Switch to the ready casserole. Press the mixture uniformly deeply into the foundation. Bake until lightly golden for 10 minutes. Put aside for coolness.

In a small heat-resistant pot, placed the boiling water. Sprinkle the gelatine with a whisk to remove the gelatine.

To smooth the cream cheese, stevia, cooled coffee and vanilla, use electric beaters in a large cup. Beat until well mixed in the gelatin mix. Fold the whipped cream. Fold. Pour the mixture on the cooled base and smooth the surface with a spatula. Cover and put for 4 hours or until placed in the refrigerator.

Using a sharp knife to cut a 16 square slice. Add extra whipped cream and coffee beans, if available. Serve with cacao dusted.

SUNDAY
BREAKFAST
Keto strawberry cheesecake balls
INGREDIENTS

- 350g strawberries, hulled
- 250g pkt cream cheese, at room temperature, chopped
- One tablespoon xylitol (see note)
- 35g (1/3 cup) desiccated coconut, plus one tablespoon, extra
- 45g (1/3 cup) pecans, finely chopped

METHOD

Preheat oven forced to 180C/160C fan. Fill a bakery tray with pastry paper.

Book 2 medium strawberries. Cut the rest of the strawberries into quarters (or sixths when large) and place them on the prepared tray. Bake for 10 minutes or until tender. Using a fork to flatten each bit slightly. Bake for another 20 minutes, or until very warm, stirring halfway. Bake for the remaining ten minutes. Switch to a plate and refresh completely.

Using electric beaters in a large bowl to mix cream cheese, strawberry pulp and xylitol. Remove the cocoa and blend together. Cover and put for 1 hour or until firm in the refrigerator.

Fill a bakery tray with pastry paper. Cut the reserved strawberries half-long, then cut into quarters every second. Take a tablespoonful of the cooled cheesecake mix and place in the middle a slice of fresh strawberry. Roll in a ball and placed on the ready tray. Repeat with remaining strawberry and mixture.

In a dish put the extra coconut and in another one the chopped pecan. Roll half of the balls in pecan and the other half in coco, slightly pushed on to cover. Place and chill in the refrigerator until strong. Store in an airtight container for up to 2 days in the refrigerator.

LUNCH
Keto garlic bread
INGREDIENTS

- 7g sachet instant dried yeast
- One tablespoon pouring cream
- 80ml (1/3 cup) warm water
- 155g (1 1/2 cups) almond meal
- Two tablespoons psyllium husk
- One tablespoon ground flaxseed
- One teaspoon baking powder
- 1/2 teaspoon table salt
- Three eggs, lightly whisked
- Two tablespoons olive oil
- Two teaspoons apple cider vinegar
- Three garlic cloves, finely chopped
- Two tablespoons olive oil
- 100g (1 cup) shredded mozzarella cheese
- Chopped continental parsley, to serve

METHOD

Grate a 20 cm square cake pot with bakery paper. In a small bowl, put the yeast, cream, and water. To combine whisk. Set aside for 10 minutes or slightly sparkling

Whisk almond meal, psyllium husk, flax, baking powder and salt in a big cup. Make a well in the centre. Attach the mixture of yeast, egg, olive oil and vinegar. Well to combine whisk. Move to the ready saucepan. Cover with plastic wrap and set aside for 1 hour or until the blend has slightly increased.

Preheat the oven to a forced 200C/180C fan. Bake the bread for fifteen minutes. Sprinkle with olive oil, garlic and sprinkle with milk. Bake for an additional 10 minutes, or bubble the cheese. To eat, sprinkle with parsley.

DINNER
Tikka chicken and cauliflower traybake
INGREDIENTS

- Four chicken thigh cutlets, skin on
- Four chicken drumsticks, skin on
- 120g (1/2 cup) tikka masala curry paste
- 270ml can light coconut milk
- 2 tsp. finely grated fresh ginger
- Two garlic cloves, crushed
- One red onion, cut into wedges
- One head (600g) cauliflower, cut into florets
- 400g can chickpeas, rinsed, drained
- 250g cherry tomatoes
- 120g baby spinach
- Fresh coriander sprigs, to serve
- Lime wedges, to serve
- Steamed brown rice, to serve

METHOD

In a bowl, put chicken bits. Apply half the curry paste to the skin and massage. Put in a large glass or plastic sealable jar.

Within a container, add the coconut milk, ginger, garlic and other curry paste. Delete to merge. Pour into the tub of the chicken.

Put in another big sealable glass or plastic tub, onion, cauliflower, chickpeas, and tomatoes.

Freeze containers up to 3 months until use or until night. Defrost in the refrigerator overnight.

Preheat oven forced to 200C/180C fan. In a large roasting bowl, place the contents of both containers. Toss to combine.

Toss to combine. Bake for 1 hour and 10 minutes or until the chicken is completely cooked. Attach spinach. Spinach. Cook for another five minutes or until the spinach wilts.

Serve with rice, lime and coriander.

Ketogenic meals can be varied and tasty, as you can see.

While many ketogenic diets are focused on animal products, there are a wide variety of vegetarian choices.

If you adopt a more liberal ketogenic diet, you may increase the number of carbs in this meal plan by adding a cup of berries to your breakfast or a little portion of a stuffed vegetable.

As every balanced diet, a ketogenic meal plan would contain whole grains and many low-carbon, fibre-rich vegetables.

For raise fat content of the dishes, use healthy fats including coconut oil, avocado, olive oil and butter.

CHAPTER 9:

KETO FLU, OTHER KETO SIDE EFFECTS, AND HOW TO CURE THEM

Now you have started a keto diet happily and look forward to many benefits. It's been a few days, though, and now you're feeling bad. You're tired, you have pain, you're easily frustrated, and you find it difficult to focus. Congratulations, you've got what is generally called keto flu. It's not exactly a fever, nor is it contagious or harmful, but it can certainly be really unpleasant. In the first one or two weeks of a keto diet, many experiences one or more of these symptoms, particularly in days 3-5. It's brief, thankfully, and soon you'll feel good again. Finally, you will have more energy than before you began your diet. Better still, a quick treatment usually alleviates most or all of these symptoms within 15 minutes. Start reading to learn more about this and other keto flu remedies!

The keto flu Symptoms of the keto flu:

- Lack of motivation
- Dizziness
- Sugar cravings
- Irritability
- Difficulty focusing ("brain fog")
- Nausea
- Fatigue
- Headache
- Muscle cramps

THE CAUSE

The keto flu happens as the body moves from the oxidation of sugar to burning fat for much of its energy needs.

The move from a high carbon diet to a very low carbon diet lowers the body's insulin levels, one of the main goals of a ketogenic diet.

If insulin levels are very small, the liver begins to turn fat into ketones, which can be used in most the cells instead of glucose. When your body uses ketones and fat primarily for energy, you are in ketosis.

Your brain and other organs will take some time to adapt to this new air. When your insulin levels go down, the body interacts with water to excrete more sodium in the urine. Regardless of this, you will probably find that in the first week or so you urinate a lot more often.

One of the swift – and often very welcome – is responsible for this change! – Loss of weight in the early stages of a keto diet. However, many of the disagreeable symptoms of keto flu are due to the loss of a lot of water and sodium.

The answer to the keto transition is well known to be very individual. Some people can feel okay or rather exhausted for a day or two after they start. At the other extreme, people develop symptoms that have a strong impact on their ability to function for several days.

Nonetheless, if appropriate steps are taken to mitigate it, keto flu will not be intolerable to everyone.

THE CURE FOR THE KETO FLU

Keto flu symptoms typically resolve within a couple of days or weeks as the body adjusts. But why not fix the cause and feel better right now instead of struggling needlessly during this time? The first step is by far the most critical, and sometimes everything is needed.

1. Increase your salt and water intake

Since the loss of salt and water is the cause of most keto-flu issues, increasing your consumption will substantially minimize and remove the symptoms.

In the first few weeks of your lifestyle, you drink a glass of water with half a teaspoon of salt when you experience headache, lethargy, nausea, dizziness or other symptoms.

Within 15 to 30 minutes, this simple action can ease your keto flu symptoms. If required, feel free to do so twice a day or more.

Or for a delicious substitute, stir in a salted butter spoon, if you prefer, drink consume, broth, bone broth, chicken stock or beef stock. And add a pinch and two of salt if you use low-sodium bone broth or stock.

Also, make sure you drink plenty of water. The heavier you are, the more water you are likely to lose in the early stages of Keto, and the more water you need to replace. It is a safe idea to drink at least 2, 5 litres of fluid each day in your first keto week. In comparison to your other drinks, you need not drink at least 2, 5 litres of plain water. Although it is important to drink lots of water, coffee and tea can also contribute to your fluid intake. However, aim to keep the intake of caffeine small (about 3 cups of coffee a day), as high levels of sodium and water will potentially increase. Adequate water, sodium and other electrolytes, such as magnesium and potassium, which can help people sometimes develop constipation in the early stages of a keto diet.

2. More fat = fewer symptoms

Through salt and fluid intakes typically overcome most side effects of the keto flu. But if you continue to feel poorly after following these recommendations, try to eat fat.

Because of decades of fat myths, fat phobias are popular among people who are new to low carbohydrates. But if you slash carbohydrates sharply without elevating your fat intake, your body would feel starving. You're going to feel tired, starving and miserable.

A well-balanced diet has enough fat to ensure you don't starve after a meal; you can go without food for many hours and have plenty of energy. At the beginning of your journey, make sure you maximize your consumption of fat until you are transitioning to the use of fat and ketones for much of your energy requirements. When you have adjusted fat, let your appetite guide you a little fat and see how comfortable you will feel. In short: Add butter or other fat to your food if in doubt. See our top ten tips to boost the intake of fat. You can also follow our keto recipes with enough fat for carbs and protein.

3. Slower transition

Has it not helped much to add more water, salt and fat? Were you both tired and sore?

We recommend that you continue to eat before symptoms pass for a few more days. Research suggests that a relatively low carbon diet is better suited to weight loss and metabolic issues such as type 2 diabetes. Keto flu effects are mild – they're going to be gone for good until you're a fat burner.

However, you can slow down the transition to ketogenic food by eating some more carbohydrates like a moderately low-carb diet that provides between 20 and 50 grams of carbon per day.

Eating a little more carbohydrates can reduce weight loss and lead to less rapid and drastic improvements in health. It can, however, still lead to better health, especially if you cut sugar and refined foods out. So keto flu won't be a problem anymore.

When you have adapted to low-carb food, consider eating less than 20 grams more to see if your body likes this or slightly higher intake of carbohydrates.

4. Take it easy with physical activity

While many people use their strength and endurance to change a keto diet, attempting to do too much can exacerbate the symptoms of keto flu.

Well-known ketogenic researcher Dr Steve Phinney carried out experiments in endurance athletes and obese adults that showed physical performance reductions in a very low-carb diet within the first week. His work shows, happily, that performance typically recovers – and frequently improves – within 4 to 6 weeks.

Walking, stretching, or doing gentle yoga or another exercise should be all right and will also make you feel better. But when your body is under stress as you begin to adjust to a new fuel system, don't burden it with any sort of punishing exercise. Taking it easy for the first few weeks and gradually through the speed of your preparation.

5. Don't consciously restrict food intake

Many people complain that the first week of Keto they are not really hungry because they have headache or nausea that reduces their appetite. Many, however, may get pretty hungry and fear that they consume too many calories to achieve their quick loss of weight.

The Atkins diet starts with induction, its strictest step, which allows for maximum fat intake and rapid entry into ketosis. With this diet, you can eat the most food you like, as long as carbs are limited to 20 or fewer grams a day.

It's not a smart idea to focus on calories as you want to adapt. When you are hungry or stressed the amount of food you consume could also worsen keto flu symptoms. If you are continually in ketosis, your appetite will possibly decline, and you will end up eating less naturally.

Drink as much of the food as possible, so you are no longer hungry and have keto snacks such as hard-boiled eggs for healthy hunger attacks. At the other side, ensure that you do not get too full by feeding slowly and paying attention to signs of hunger and fullness.

CHAPTER 10:

INTERMITTENT FASTING ON THE KETO DIET

Everyone wants to be the healthiest person they can be, and obviously, you're no exception. Unfortunately, it's difficult to tell if a strategy to lose weight or improve wellbeing is real or just a bunch of smoke and mirrors with too many fad diets and too much bad advice.

Many rely on superfoods to find the best time to feed, leading to multiple questions.

One popular question is also one of the biggest we saw: Could you do intermittent fasting and keto simultaneously?

WHAT IS KETO?

Someone who has been in the world of diet, wellness and nutrition for a short period is probably aware of the keto diet.

This was the last craze a couple of years ago, and since then it has just seemed to become more popular.

Why? Because it works.

The keto diet is a special diet, which basically excludes carbs while concentrating on the appropriate fat and protein type. This does not completely remove carbohydrates but focuses on entering a ketosis state.

During ketosis, the body hits a specific fat-burning high and uses all of its additional stocks throughout the body to help a person lose excessively and excessive fat.

The Keto diet provides many nutritional benefits and supports people with mental conditions and illnesses such as Alzheimer's. Several positive factors include lowered blood sugar, increased insulin tolerance and even lower heart disease factors.

The keto diet can at first seem overwhelming but is really a great way to remove empty calories from carbohydrates, which have little to no nutrition.

WHAT IS INTERMITTENT FASTING?

Most people are scared when they see the term 'fasting' as it is synonymous with poverty and hunger.

But when someone has intermittent fasting, they don't hunger or hurt their bodies.

Rather, they limit the window where they take calories to help the body even out.

Somebody who eats only eight hours on the window during the day and doesn't eat for the remaining sixteen hours would be an example of an intermittent fast. This is referred to as the 16/8 method.

It ensures that the body gets daily nutrients, but does not flood its systems in the form of calories with unneeded energy.

Some people use 5:2 or alternate-day fasting more extreme, but this is not necessary to lose weight.

Intermittent quicking is perfectly healthy when correct and has been done by people for thousands of years. Monks often fast, some religions have whole days around fasting, and people eat only every other day.

This method also has health benefits such as lower blood sugar and less resistance to insulin. It can also reduce inflammation, improve brain function and even eliminate day-to-day leniency due to contemporary lifestyles.

Why wouldn't want to be more vigorous?

ARE THEY SAFE TOGETHER?

In short, yes, it is safe to fast and keto simultaneously. The trick is to ensure that you get enough nutrients and calories to keep functioning while you still go ketosis.

Throughout ketosis, the body is produced throughout fat-burning mode and feasts on all the additional stores that build up throughout the body.

Keto removes excessive sugar from your diet, and you can conveniently consume all of your required vitamins, minerals, proteins and healthy fats.

By combining keto with a simple 16/8 intermittent quick, you ensure that your body gets its nutrients while still eliminating fat cells.

The trick is to concentrate your keto diet only on the right things. So eat plenty of lean, red, and dark, leafy protein.

There are possible drawbacks of mixing IF and keto.

Second, recognize that Keto focuses primarily on weight loss rather than on overall health and that intermittent fasting doesn't change this. When you do it incorrectly, Keto can be dangerous, despite mixing it with when.

For example, a diet of ketones, which is mostly butter and bacon, is different from an olive oil and avocado diet. A poorly planned keto diet with IF can lead to nutritional deficiencies because intermittent fasting reduces calories significantly.

Athletic success may also be impaired by mixing keto and intermittent fasting. So, if you're in sports, your game performance could be very successful in combining the two dietary methods.

In addition, this combination is riskier for some than for others. The easiest way to stop mixing keto and intermittent fasting are for the following people:

Girls who are pregnant and breastfeeding. Many new mothers may be looking forward to weighing the infant, but producing milk takes considerable energy.

Children under the age of 18 years. The rising age is where they can eat if they want to eat.

Men over the age of 65. We are likely to find it difficult to get enough calories and nutrients as they are.

People with nutritional deficiency and others who need food for their medicines.

Individuals with or now have an eating disorder.

Persons with other conditions of health, such as heart disease or diabetes, should consult with a doctor before fasting.

BENEFITS

Thanks to many additional characteristics, Keto and intermittent fasting work exceptionally well together and also provide a wide variety of specific health benefits.

Intermittent fasting shortens the time to get into ketosis

Ketosis is a normal condition of the body that occurs not only when the body starts to use fat to produce energy, including fasting and exercise, but also on a low-carb diet. Most people are ketosised while fasting, so extending their time between meals will help them get into ketosis more easily.

Promotes weight loss

Intermittent fasting and the keto diet encourage your body to use fat instead of glucose for energy. The combination of intermittent fasting with a keto diet, therefore, improves your weight loss.

Creates a caloric deficit

The quick look removes at least one meal from your day, potentially leading to a caloric deficit — a key component of weight loss (except if you make up for more calories during the calories fan).

Reduces your appetite by making fasting easier

Replacing fat carbs on a keto diet leads to decreased appetite, possibly because of changes in appetite regulation hormones.

After you have a fat-fitting diet and an appetite lower than normal, the quicking portion of intermittent fasting will be easier to find.

HOW TO DO INTERMITTENT FASTING ON KETO 7 STEPS TO GET STARTED

STEP 1:

EASE INTO INTERMITTENT FASTING

The best way to begin intermittent fasting is to promote an intermittent fasting lifestyle.

If you are a complete beginner to fast, start with intermittent fasting for 16/8 days without changing your diet.

When you have experience with fasting and are positive about it, you should go straight ahead and make dietary adjustments.

Our 21-day Fasting Challenge Program recommends slowly rising you're eating window to help your body adjust to irregular quickness. In other words, on the first day, you start with 12 hours quickly and slowly increasing it to 16 hours.

Where do you pick your quick / eat window? To most people, breakfast is the best, but some people prefer to spend dinner instead. Few scenarios for an intermittent diet of 16/8 keto:

- If you start eating at 12 pm, start fasting at 8 pm
- If you start eating at 2 pm stop eating and start fasting at 10 pm
- If you start eating at 8 am, start fasting at 4 pm

STEP 2:

INTRODUCE A KETO DIET: WHAT TO EAT?

Feel good to stick to your sporadic schedule? Great! Great! Your next move is a ketogenic diet to change your eating. Decide if you adopt the keto diet – either by adhering to a 5/70/25 macro nutritional breakdown or by using net carbohydrates only. Here is a list of foods for an intermittent fasting diet recommended for keto.

KETO INTERMITTENT FASTING FRIENDLY FOODS Foods with little or no-carb per cent, like:

- Green and leafy vegetables
- Unprocessed meat such as beef, pork, lamb, poultry
- Eggs
- Berries (in moderation).
- High-fat fish like salmon, mackerel, sardines
- Butter and full-fat dairy products
- Oils
- Nuts such as pecan, brazil, macadamia

FOODS NOT ALLOWED ON KETO INTERMITTENT FASTING

Grains and starches: wheat, rice, rye, corn, quinoa, buckwheat, bulgur

Grain products: pasta, bread, cereal, oatmeal, pastries, muesli, pizza

Legumes: beans, chickpeas, lentils, peas

Root vegetables: potato, sweet potato, parsnip, yam

Most fruits

Sugar and sweetened products such as sauces, soda, juice.

You can also restrict the intake of certain fruits, dairy products, nuts and seeds to ensure that you stay within the necessary macro limits.

STEP 3:

HOW TO CALCULATE NET CARBS?

You may have learned that carbs are not the same. Remember that for the keto diet, net carbs matter in comparison to total carbohydrates.

What are the net carbs that you are looking for? Net carbs are the cumulative sum of carbs that your body consumes. Fibre, which exists naturally in most whole foods, moves directly to the colon and is thus removed for net carbs.

Check their nutritional value online for unpackaged and unprocessed foods such as vegetables,fruits, nuts, meat and other products.

Net carbs are measured by subtracting the fibres from the total carbs for packaged goods with a Nutritional Facts mark.

STEP 4:

HOW TO REACH KETOSIS?

Eating a low-carb diet will automatically help the body go into ketosis. With the reduction in carbon intake, much less glucose is produced. This transforms your body from the use of glucose as energy to the burning of stored fat.

Fatter intake is as important as reducing carbohydrates. The fat from food supports and maintains ketone production.

Enough protein to feed. Protein should not become the main component of your diet, however, because it allows the body to become gluconeo genetic. Gluconeogenesis kicks you out of ketosis because the body produces protein glucose.

Ketosis should occur between 12 hours and seven days after an intermittent fasting diet starts.

STEP 5:

YOUR TYPICAL DAY ON KETO INTERMITTENT FASTING

Wonder how a typical meal day on an intermittent fasting schedule looks?

Below is a 16/8 fasting form, but you can typically adapt it to your preference.

8 am: Cup of black coffee or tea

12:00 noon: Chicken breast with avocado oil, served with buttery sautéed spinach

3-3:30 pm: Keto chia seed and flax seed pudding with strawberries

7-8 pm: Baked salmon with dill, with cooked asparagus, butter, parmesan, and sliced almonds

STEP 6:

HOW TO TEST IF YOU ARE IN KETOSIS?

Since our bodies are special, ketosis may be achieved before another. You may select one of three ways to test reliably whether you have achieved ketosis and to assess your ketone levels:

- Through urine using keto strips
- Through blood analysis
- Through a simple breath using ketone breath analyzers.

Although daily blood is too difficult and expensive, urine strips and breathing analyzers provide easy solutions at home.

Personally, we prefer the accuracy and simplicity of breath ketone monitors to both options. These are easy to use on the go (no need to hurry to the bathroom while working and/or carrying test kits) and allow the quality of your diet to be checked as many times as you like.

STEP 7:

WHO IS KETO INTERMITTENT FASTING NOT FOR?

The last thing is to do before you go and decide to make intermittent fasting, to know that it's a good choice for you. While it is usually safe for most healthy people, some people should avoid intermittent fasting, especially:

- if you take medications for blood pressure or heart disease
- if you are pregnant or breastfeeding
- if you have a history of disordered eating
- if you don't sleep well
- If you are under 18 years old.

Needless to say, if you have any issues or are uncertain, your doctor will always determine if Keto Intermittent Fasting is healthy for you and how long you can. The important thing to note is that a low carb diet for a longer period of time is not recommended. It's a perfect way to boost weight loss and improve your health, but it does not encourage a healthy lifestyle forever.

CHAPTER 11:

BREAKFAST

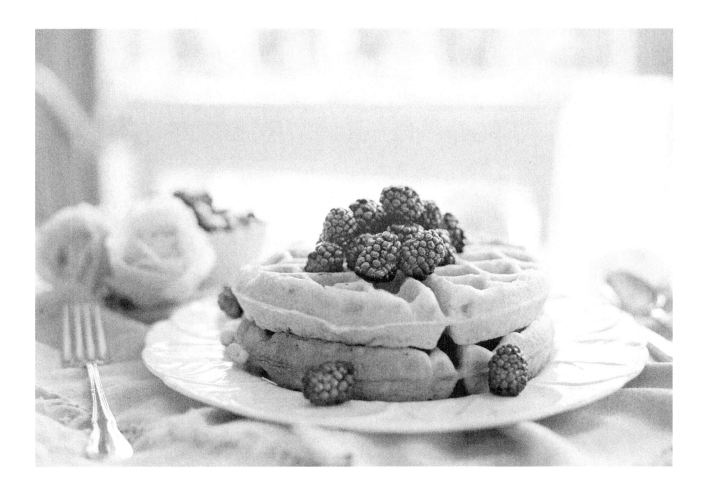

ALMOND FLOUR PANCAKES

Preparation Time: 5 minutes
Cooking Time: 5 minutes
Servings: 4
Ingredients

- ½ cup almond flour
- ½ cup cream cheese
- 4 medium eggs
- ½ tsp cinnamon
- ½ tsp granulated sweetener
- 1 tsp grass-fed butter
- 1 tbsp sugar-free syrup

Directions

1. Add all the ingredients into a blender and let them blend in well. Once done, set the batter aside.
2. On a non-stick pan at medium heat, fry pancakes with melted butter. Once the center starts to bubble, turn over. Once done with the pancake, move on to the rest, using the batter.
3. Finally, serve your pancakes warm, along with some low carb fruit or with an exquisite side of sugar-free syrup to enjoy a healthy and tasty breakfast.

Nutrition:
Calories: 234
Fat: 20g
Carbohydrates: 4g
Fiber: 1.5g
Net carbs: 2.5g
Protein: 11g

AVOCADO TOAST

Preparation Time: 20 minutes
Cooking Time: 40 minutes
Servings: 2
Ingredients

- ½ cup grass-fed butter
- 2 tbsp coconut oil
- 7 large eggs
- 1 tsp baking powder
- 2 cups almond flour
- ½ tsp xanthan gum
- ½ tsp kosher salt
- 1 medium avocado

Directions

1. Preheat over at 3500F. Beat eggs for around two minutes with a mixer at high speed. Then, add coconut oil and butter (both melted) to the eggs and continue beating. Ensure that oil and butter are not too warm to cook the eggs. Add remaining bread ingredients and mix well. Now, the batter should become thick. Pour batter in a non-stick loaf pan lined with parchment paper. Let it bake for 45 minutes or until the fork comes clean through the middle.
2. For topping, toast two slices of your keto bread to your liking. Slice the whole avocado thinly, without the skin or pit. Use these to make one long strip of overlapping slices. Roll these into a spiral and that is it! Enjoy your keto bread with avocado topping.

Nutrition:
Calories: 350 Fat: 32g Carbohydrates: 7g
Fiber: 4g Net carbs: 3g Protein: 10g

CHICKEN AVOCADO EGG BACON SALAD

Preparation Time: 10 minutes
Cooking Time: 10 minutes
Servings: 4
Ingredients

- 12 oz. cooked chicken breast
- 6 slices crumbled bacon
- 3 boiled eggs cut into cubes
- 1 cup cherry tomatoes cut into halves
- 1/2 small sliced red onion
- 1 large avocado(s)
- 1/2 stick finely chopped celery
- Salad Dressing
- 1/2 cup olive oil mayonnaise
- 2 tbsp. sour cream
- 1 tsp Dijon mustard
- 4 tbsp. extra virgin olive oil
- 2 cloves minced garlic
- 2 tsp lemon juice
- 4 cups lettuce
- Salt and pepper to taste

Directions

1. Combine all the ingredients together and mix them well for the salad dressing. Then, combine chicken, tomatoes, bacon, eggs, red onions, and celery together. Add about ¾ of the salad dressing and mix them well. Add the avocado and toss together gently. Check the taste and, if needed, add the remainder of the salad dressing as well. Finally, add salt and pepper to taste and then serve it over lettuce.

Nutrition:
Calories: 387 Fat: 27g Carbohydrates: 2.5g
Fiber: 1g Net carbs: 1.5g Protein: 24g

BACON WRAPPED CHICKEN BREAST

Preparation Time: 10 minutes
Cooking Time: 45 minutes
Servings: 4
Ingredients

- 4 boneless, skinless chicken breast
- 8 oz. sharp cheddar cheese
- 8 slices bacon
- 4 oz. sliced jalapeno peppers
- 1 tsp garlic powder
- Salt and pepper to taste

Directions

1. Preheat the oven at around 3500F. Ensure to season both sides of chicken breast well with salt, garlic powder, and pepper. Place the chicken breast on a non-stick baking sheet (foil-covered). Cover the chicken with cheese and add jalapeno slices. Cut the bacon slices in half and then place the four halves over each piece of chicken. Bake for around 30 to 45 minutes at most. If the chicken is set but the bacon still feels undercooked, you may want to put it under the broiler for a few minutes. Once done, serve hot with a side of low carb garlic parmesan roasted asparagus.

Nutrition:
Calories: 640 Fat: 48g
Carbohydrates: 6g Fiber: 3g
Net carbs: 3g Protein: 47g

EGG SALAD

Preparation Time: 15 minutes
Cooking Time: 10 minutes
Servings: 4
Ingredients

- 6 eggs
- 2 tbsp mayonnaise
- 1 tsp Dijon mustard
- 1 tsp lemon juice
- Salt and pepper to taste

Directions

1. In a medium saucepan, place the solid eggs gently.
2. Add some cold water so that the eggs are covered around an inch. Boil them for around 10 minutes.
3. Once done, remove them from the heat and let them cool. Peel the eggs while running them under cold water. Now add these in a food processor and pulse until they are chopped.
4. Add and stir mayonnaise, lemon juice, mustard, and salt and pepper. Ensure to taste and then adjust as necessary.
5. Finally, serve them with a bit of lettuce leaves and, if needed, bacon for wrapping.

Nutrition:
Calories: 222 Fat: 19g
Net carbs: 1g
Protein: 13g

BLUEBERRY MUFFINS

Preparation Time: 10 minutes
Cooking Time: 30 minutes
Servings: 12
Ingredients

- 1 container Greek yogurt
- 3 large eggs
- 1/2 tsp vanilla extract
- 1/4 tsp salt
- 2 1/2 cups almond flour
- 1/4 cup Swerve sweetener (add more if using plain Greek yogurt)
- 2 tsp baking powder
- Water if needed to thin
- 1/2 cup fresh blueberries

Directions

1. Preheat oven at 325°F. Simultaneously, line-up a clean muffin pan with around 12 parchment liners. Combine yogurt, vanilla, eggs, and salt in a blender. Blend the mixture till it is smooth. Add almond flour, baking powder and sweetener. Now, blend again until it is smooth. If the batter is thick, add one tablespoon of water at a time. The batter should be thick, but it must be pourable.
2. Add in blueberries and divide these equally for the prepared muffin cups. Finally, bake these for 25 to 30 minutes. Use a tester and insert it right in the middle. If it comes out clean, your muffins are ready.

Nutrition:
Calories: 163 Net carbs: 3.8g
Fat: 12.9g
Protein: 7.6g

BACON HASH

Preparation Time: 5 minutes
Cooking Time: 10 minutes
Servings: 2
Ingredients:

- Small green pepper (1)
- Jalapenos (2)
- Small onion (1)
- Eggs (4)
- Bacon slices (6)

Directions:

1. Chop the bacon into chunks using a food processor. Set aside for now. Slice the onions and peppers into thin strips. Dice the jalapenos as small as possible.
2. Heat a skillet and fry the veggies. Once browned, combine the fixings and cook until crispy. Place on a serving dish with the eggs.

Nutrition:
Carbohydrates: 9 grams
Protein: 23 grams
Fats: 24 grams
Calories: 366

BAGELS WITH CHEESE

Preparation Time: 10 minutes
Cooking Time: 15 minutes
Servings: 6
Ingredients:

- Mozzarella cheese (2.5 cups)
- Baking powder (1 tsp.)
- Cream cheese (3 oz.)
- Almond flour (1.5 cups)
- Eggs (2)

Directions:

1. Shred the mozzarella and combine with the flour, baking powder, and cream cheese in a mixing container. Pop into the microwave for about one minute. Mix well.
2. Let the mixture cool and add the eggs. Break apart into six sections and shape into round bagels. Note: You can also sprinkle with a seasoning of your choice or pinch of salt if desired.
3. Bake them for approximately 12 to 15 minutes. Serve or cool and store.

Nutrition:
Carbohydrates: 8 grams
Protein: 19 grams Fats: 31 grams
Calories: 374

CAULI FLITTERS

Preparation Time: 10 minutes
Cooking Time: 15 minutes
Servings: 2
Ingredients:

- 2 eggs
- 1 head of cauliflower
- 1 tbsp. yeast
- sea salt, black pepper
- 1-2 tbsp. ghee
- 1 tbsp. turmeric
- 2/3 cup almond flour

Directions:
1. Place the cauliflower into a large pot and start to boil it for 8 mins. Add the florets into a food processor and pulse them.
2. Add the eggs, almond flour, yeast, turmeric, salt and pepper to a mixing bowl. Stir well. Form into patties.
3. Heat your ghee to medium in a skillet. Form your fritters and cook until golden on each side (3-4 mins).
4. Serve it while hot.

Nutrition:
Calories: 238 kcal Fat: 23 g
Carbs: 5 g Protein: 6 g

SCRAMBLED EGGS

Preparation Time: 2 minutes
Cooking Time: 8 minutes
Servings: 4
Ingredients:
- 4 oz. butter
- 8 eggs
- salt and pepper for taste

Directions:
1. Crack the eggs in a bowl, and whisk them together, while seasoning it.
2. Melt the butter in a skillet over medium heat, but don't turn it into brown.
3. Pour the eggs into the skillet and cook it for 1-2 mins, until they look and feel fluffy and creamy.
4. Tip: If you want to shake things up, you can pair this one up with bacon, salmon, or maybe avocado as well.

Nutrition:
Carbs: 1 g Fat: 31 g
Protein: 11 g
Calories: 327 kcal

FRITTATA WITH SPINACH

Preparation Time: 5 minutes
Cooking Time: 30 minutes
Servings: 4
Ingredients:
- 8 eggs
- 8 ozs. fresh spinach
- 5 ozs. diced bacon
- 5 ozs. shredded cheese
- 1 cup heavy whipping cream
- 2 tbsps. butter
- salt and pepper

Directions:
1. Preheat the oven to 350 °F
2. Fry the bacon until crispy, add the spinach and cook until wilted. Set them aside.
3. Whisk the cream and eggs together, and pour it into the baking dish.
4. Add the cheese, spinach, and bacon on the top, and place in the oven. Bake for 25-30 minutes, until golden brown on top.

Nutrition:
Carbs: 4 g
Fat: 59 g
Protein: 27 g
Calories: 661 kcal

CHEESE OMELET

Preparation Time: 5 minutes
Cooking Time: 10 minutes
Servings: 2
Ingredients:
- 6 eggs
- 3 ozs. ghee
- 7 ozs. shredded cheddar cheese
- salt and pepper

Directions:
1. Whisk the eggs until smooth. Compound half of the cheese and season it with salt and pepper.
2. Melt the butter in a pan. Pour in the mixture and let it sit for a few minutes (3-4)
3. When the mixture is looking good, add the other half of the cheese. Serve immediately.

Nutrition:
Carbs: 4 g Fat: 80 g Protein: 40 g Calories: 897 kcal

CAPICOLA EGG CUPS

Preparation Time: 5 minutes
Cooking Time: 15 minutes
Servings: 4
Ingredients:
- 8 eggs
- 1 cup cheddar cheese
- 4 oz. capicola or bacon (slices)
- salt, pepper, basil

Directions:
1. Preheat the oven to 400°F. You will need 8 wells of a standard-size muffin pan.
2. Place the slices in the 8 wells, forming a cup shape. Sprinkle into each cup some of the cheese, according to your liking.
3. Crack an egg into each cup, season them with salt and pepper.
4. Bake for 10-15 mins. Serve hot, top it with basil.

Nutrition:
Carbs: 1 g Fat: 11 g
Protein: 16 g
Calories: 171 kcal

OVERNIGHT "NOATS"

Preparation Time: 5 minutes plus overnight to chill
Cooking Time: 10 minutes
Servings: 1
Ingredients:
- 2 tablespoons hulled hemp seeds
- 1 tablespoon chia seeds
- ½ scoop (about 8 grams) collagen powder
- ½ cup unsweetened nut or seed milk (hemp, almond, coconut, and cashew)

Direction:
1. In a small mason jar or glass container, combine the hemp seeds, chia seeds, collagen, and milk.
2. Secure tightly with a lid, shake well, and refrigerate overnight.

Nutrition:
Calories: 263 Total Fat: 19g Protein: 16g
Total Carbs: 7g Fiber: 5g
Net Carbs: 2g

FROZEN KETO COFFEE

Preparation Time: 5 minutes
Cooking Time: 20 minutes
Servings: 1
Ingredients:

- 12 ounces coffee, chilled
- 1 scoop MCT powder (or 1 tablespoon MCT oil)
- 1 tablespoon heavy (whipping) cream
- Pinch ground cinnamon
- Dash sweetener (optional)
- ½ cup ice

Directions:

1. In a blender, combine the coffee, MCT powder, cream, cinnamon, sweetener (if using), and ice. Blend until smooth.

Nutrition:
Calories: 127; Total Fat: 13g;
Protein: 1g; Total Carbs: 1.5g; Fiber: 1g; Net Carbs: 0.5g

EASY SKILLET PANCAKES

Preparation Time: 5 minutes
Cooking Time: 5 minutes
Servings: 8
Ingredients:

- 8 ounces cream cheese- 8 eggs
- 2 tablespoons coconut flour
- 2 teaspoons baking powder
- 1 teaspoon ground cinnamon
- ½ teaspoon vanilla extract
- 1 teaspoon liquid stevia or sweetener of choice (optional)
- 2 tablespoons butter

Directions

1. In a blender, combine the cream cheese, eggs, coconut flour, baking powder, cinnamon, vanilla, and stevia (if using). Blend until smooth.
2. In a large skillet over medium heat, melt the butter.
3. Use half the mixture to pour four evenly sized pancakes and cook for about a minute, until you see bubbles on top. Flip the pancakes and cook for another minute. Remove from the pan and add more butter or oil to the skillet if needed. Repeat with the remaining batter.
4. Top with butter and eat right away, or freeze the pancakes in a freezer-safe resealable bag with sheets of parchment in between, for up to 1 month.

Nutrition:
Calories: 179 Total Fat: 15g
Protein: 8g Total Carbs: 3g Fiber: 1g Net Carbs: 2g

QUICK KETO BLENDER MUFFINS

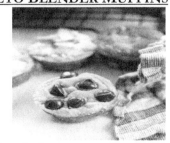

Preparation Time: 5 minutes
Cooking Time: 25 minutes
Servings: 12

Ingredients

- Butter, ghee, or coconut oil for greasing the pan
- 6 eggs
- 8 ounces cream cheese, at room temperature
- 2 scoops flavored collagen powder
- 1 teaspoon ground cinnamon
- 1 teaspoon baking powder
- Few drops or dash sweetener (optional)

Directions:

1. Preheat the oven to 350ºF. Grease a 12-cup muffin pan very well with butter, ghee, or coconut oil. Alternatively, you can use silicone cups or paper muffin liners.
2. In a blender, combine the eggs, cream cheese, collagen powder, cinnamon, baking powder, and sweetener (if using). Blend until well combined and pour the mixture into the muffin cups, dividing equally.
3. Bake for 22 to 25 minutes until the muffins are golden brown on top and firm.
4. Let cool then store in a glass container or plastic bag in the refrigerator for up to 2 weeks or in the freezer for up to 3 months.
5. To Servings refrigerated muffins, heat in the microwave for 30 seconds. To Servings from frozen, thaw in the refrigerator overnight and then microwave for 30 seconds, or microwave straight from the freezer for 45 to 60 seconds or until heated through.

Nutrition:
Calories: 120 Total Fat: 10g
Protein: 6g Total Carbs: 1.5g
Fiber: 0g
Net Carbs: 1.5g

KETO EVERYTHING BAGELS

Preparation Time: 10 minutes
Cooking Time: 15 minutes
Servings: 8
Ingredients:

- 2 cups shredded mozzarella cheese
- 2 tablespoons labneh cheese (or cream cheese)
- 1½ cups almond flour
- 1 egg
- 2 teaspoons baking powder
- ¼ teaspoon sea salt
- 1 tablespoon

Directions

1. Preheat the oven to 400ºF.
2. In a microwave-safe bowl, combine the mozzarella and labneh cheeses. Microwave for 30 seconds, stir, then microwave for another 30 seconds. Stir well. If not melted completely, microwave for another 10 to 20 seconds.
3. Add the almond flour, egg, baking powder, and salt to the bowl and mix well. Form into a dough using a spatula or your hands.
4. Cut the dough into 8 roughly equal pieces and form into balls.
5. Roll each dough ball into a cylinder, then pinch the ends together to seal.
6. Place the dough rings in a nonstick donut pan or arrange them on a parchment paper–lined baking sheet.
7. Sprinkle with the seasoning and bake for 12 to 15 minutes or until golden brown.

8. Store in plastic bags in the freezer and defrost overnight in the refrigerator. Reheat in the oven or toaster for a quick grab-and-go breakfast.

Nutrition:
Calories: 241
Total Fat: 19g
Protein: 12g
Total Carbs: 5.5g
Fiber: 2.5g
Net Carbs: 3g

TURMERIC CHICKEN AND KALE SALAD WITH FOOD, LEMON AND HONEY

Preparation Time: 20 minutes
Cooking Time: 15 minutes
Servings: 4
Ingredients:
- For the chicken:
- 1 teaspoon of clarified butter or 1 tablespoon of coconut oil
- ½ medium brown onion, diced
- 250-300 g / 9 ounces minced chicken meat or diced chicken legs
- 1 large garlic clove, diced
- 1 teaspoon of turmeric powder
- 1 teaspoon of lime zest
- ½ lime juice
- ½ teaspoon of salt + pepper
- For the salad:
- 6 stalks of broccoli or 2 cups of broccoli flowers
- 2 tablespoons of pumpkin seeds (seeds)
- 3 large cabbage leaves, stems removed and chopped
- ½ sliced avocado
- Handful of fresh coriander leaves, chopped
- Handful of fresh parsley leaves, chopped
- For the dressing:
- 3 tablespoons of lime juice
- 1 small garlic clove, diced or grated
- 3 tablespoons of virgin olive oil (I used 1 tablespoon of avocado oil and 2 tablespoons of EVO)
- 1 teaspoon of raw honey
- ½ teaspoon whole or Dijon mustard
- ½ teaspoon of sea salt with pepper

Directions:
1. Heat the coconut oil in a pan. Add the onion and sauté over medium heat for 4-5 minutes, until golden brown. Add the minced chicken and garlic and stir 2-3 minutes over medium-high heat, separating.
2. Add your turmeric, lime zest, lime juice, salt and pepper, and cook, stirring consistently, for another 3-4 minutes. Set the ground beef aside.
3. While your chicken is cooking, put a small saucepan of water to the boil. Add your broccoli and cook for 2 minutes. Rinse with cold water and cut into 3-4 pieces each.
4. Add the pumpkin seeds to the chicken pan and toast over medium heat for 2 minutes, frequently stirring to avoid burning. Season with a little salt. Set aside. Raw pumpkin seeds are also good to use.
5. Put the chopped cabbage in a salad bowl and pour it over the dressing. Using your hands, mix, and massage the cabbage with the dressing. This will soften the cabbage, a bit like citrus juice with fish or beef Carpaccio: it "cooks" it a little.
6. Finally, mix the cooked chicken, broccoli, fresh herbs, pumpkin seeds, and avocado slices.

Nutrition:
232 calories Fat 11 Fiber 9 Carbs 8 Protein 14

BUCKWHEAT SPAGHETTI WITH CHICKEN CABBAGE AND SAVORY FOOD RECIPES IN MASS SAUCE

Preparation Time: 15 minutes
Cooking Time: 15 minutes'
Servings: 2
Ingredients:
- For the noodles:
- 2-3 handfuls of cabbage leaves (removed from the stem and cut)
- Buckwheat noodles 150g / 5oz (100% buckwheat, without wheat)
- 3-4 shiitake mushrooms, sliced
- 1 teaspoon of coconut oil or butter
- 1 brown onion, finely chopped
- 1 medium chicken breast, sliced or diced
- 1 long red pepper, thinly sliced (seeds in or out depending on how hot you like it)
- 2 large garlic cloves, diced
- 2-3 tablespoons of Tamari sauce (gluten-free soy sauce)
- For the miso dressing:
- 1 tablespoon and a half of fresh organic miso
- 1 tablespoon of Tamari sauce
- 1 tablespoon of extra virgin olive oil
- 1 tablespoon of lemon or lime juice
- 1 teaspoon of sesame oil (optional)

Directions:
1. Boil a medium saucepan of water. Add the black cabbage and cook 1 minute, until it is wilted. Remove and reserve, but reserve the water and return to boiling. Add your soba noodles and cook according to the directions on the package (usually about 5 minutes). Rinse with cold water and reserve.
2. In the meantime, fry the shiitake mushrooms in a little butter or coconut oil (about a teaspoon) for 2-3 minutes, until its color is lightly browned on each side. Sprinkle with sea salt and reserve.
3. In that same pan, heat more coconut oil or lard over medium-high heat. Fry the onion and chili for 2-3 minutes, and then add the chicken pieces. Cook 5 minutes on medium heat, stirring a few times, then add the garlic, tamari sauce, and a little water. Cook for another 2-3 minutes, stirring continuously until your chicken is cooked.
4. Finally, add the cabbage and soba noodles and stir the chicken to warm it.
5. Stir the miso sauce and sprinkle the noodles at the end of the cooking, in this way you will keep alive all the beneficial probiotics in the miso.

Nutrition:
305 calories Fat 11
Fiber 7 Carbs 9 Protein 12

CHAPTER 12:

LUNCH

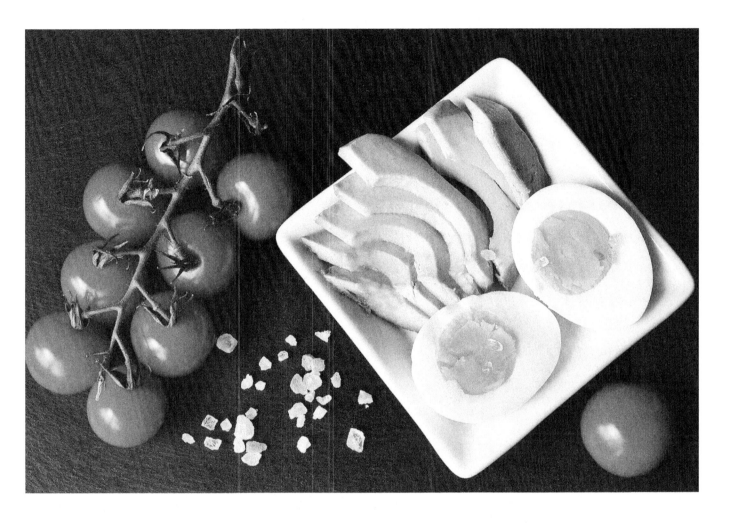

3-CHEESE CHICKEN AND CAULIFLOWER LASAGNA

INGREDIENTS

- One tablespoon extra-virgin olive oil
- One leek, trimmed, thinly sliced
- 500g chicken mince
- 200g punnet button mushrooms, sliced
- One bunch English spinach, trimmed, rinsed, dried, chopped
- 250g packet cream cheese, chopped
- One teaspoon dried tarragon
- 125ml (1/2 cup) tomato pasta sauce
- 100g (1 cup) coarsely grated mozzarella
- CAULIFLOWER LASAGNE SHEETS
- 1.1kg cauliflower, trimmed, coarsely chopped
- 40g (1/2 cup) finely grated parmesan
- Two eggs

METHOD

Process half of the cauliflower in a food processor for the lasagne cauliflower sheets until finely chopped. Switch to a secure bowl with a microwave. Repeat the rest of the cauliflower. Cover and microwave on warm, often stirring for 8-10 minutes or tenderly. Drain through a fine sieve and press with a wooden spoon until excess liquid is removed. Return to the bowl and add the egg and parmesan. Saison. Saison. Remove well to combine.

Preheat oven forced to 180C /160C fan. Line 2 big bakery trays with bakery paper. Divide the chocolate mixture between the prepared trays and use your fingertips or a pallet knife to gently push every batch of the cauliflower mixture into 22 x 30 cm rectangles. Cook until the mixture has dried up for 15-20 minutes. Put aside for coolness. Cut into 10 cm lasagne sheets (6 sheets should be available).

Meanwhile, heat the oil over high heat in a large non-stick pot. Connect the leek. Connect the leek. Reduce heat to low, stir sometimes, or until soft for 4 minutes. Temperature up to big. Add chicken and cook for 5 minutes or until cooked, breaking with a wooden spoon. Attach the champignons. Cook, often stirring, for 5 minutes or until champagne is golden. Add lettuce. Add lettuce. Cook for 4 minutes or until spinach is wilted, whisking occasionally. Add cream cheese. Add cream cheese. Cook, stir until cheese has melted for 2 minutes. Remove the tarragon and the season. Set aside. Set aside.

Grate square 19 cm (base measurement) with a bakery plate of 24 cm (top measurement). Brush the foundation with half the tomato pasta sauce gently. Layer 2 lasagne parts over the pasta sauce. Sprinkle with 1/3 cup mozzarella with half of the chicken mixture. Repeat with another cauliflower layer and chicken mixture. Cover with the rest of the lasagne. Continue with the rest of the pasta and mozzarella sauce. Bake until golden for 30 minutes. Set aside before serving for 7 minutes to rest.

AVOCADO, PROSCIUTTO AND PECAN SALAD

INGREDIENTS

- Eight slices prosciutto, thin
- Three avocados
- One tablespoon lime rind, finely grated
- 1/3 cup lime juice
- 1/4 cup extra virgin olive oil
- 1 cup fresh coriander leaves
- 1 cup fresh flat-leaf parsley leaves
- 2/3 cup pecans, toasted, roughly chopped
- Two long red chillies, seeded, finely chopped

METHOD

Place over high heat a large frying pan.

Fill in the prosciutto.

Cook for two minutes, or until golden and crisp, on each side.

Drain on a towel of paper.

Split in half.

Peel and fourteen avocados.

Placed in a cup.

Attach lime, juice and oil. Rind lime. Salt and pepper season. Pack. Gently flip to cover. Arrange avocado in a bowl to eat. Sprinkle with prosciutto, coriander, pecans, and chilli peppers.

Honor. Honor.

CHICKEN IN SWEET AND SOUR SAUCE WITH CORN SALAD

Preparation Time: 10 minutes
Cooking Time: 15 minutes
Servings: 4
Ingredients:

- 2 cups plus 2 tablespoons of unflavored low-fat yoghurt
- 2 cups of frozen mango chunks
- 3 tablespoons of honey
- ¼ cup plus 1 tablespoon apple cider vinegar
- ¼ cup sultana
- 2 tablespoons of olive oil, plus an amount to be brushed
- ¼ teaspoon of cayenne pepper
- 5 dried tomatoes (not in oil)
- 2 small cloves of garlic, finely chopped
- 4 cobs, peeled
- 8 peeled and boned chicken legs, peeled (about 700g)
- Halls
- 6 cups of mixed salad
- 2 medium carrots, finely sliced

Directions:

1. For the smoothie: in a blender, mix 2 cups of yogurt, 2 cups of ice, 1 cup of mango and all the honey until the mixture becomes completely smooth. Divide into 4 glasses and refrigerate until ready to use. Rinse the blender.

2. Preheat the grill to medium-high heat. Mix the remaining cup of mango, ¼ cup water, ¼ cup vinegar, sultanas, olive oil, cayenne pepper, tomatoes and garlic in a microwave bowl. Cover with a piece of clear film and cook in the microwave until the tomatoes become soft, for about 3

minutes. Leave to cool slightly and pass in a blender. Transfer to a small bowl. Leave 2 tablespoons aside to garnish, turn the chicken into the remaining mixture.

3. Put the corn on the grill, cover and bake, turning it over if necessary, until it is burnt, about 10 minutes. Remove and keep warm.

4. Brush the grill over medium heat and brush the grills with a little oil. Turn the chicken legs into half the remaining sauce and ½ teaspoon of salt. Put on the grill and cook until the cooking marks appear and the internal temperature reaches 75°C on an instantaneous thermometer, 8 to 10 minutes per side. Bart and sprinkle a few times with the remaining sauce while cooking.

5. While the chicken is cooking, beat the remaining 2 tablespoons of yogurt, the 2 tablespoons of sauce set aside, the remaining spoonful of vinegar, 1 tablespoon of water and ¼ teaspoon of salt in a large bowl. Mix the mixed salad with the carrots. Divide chicken, corn and salad into 4 serving dishes. Garnish the salad with the dressing set aside. Serve each plate with a mango smoothie.

Nutrition:
Calories 346
Protein 56
Fat 45

CHINESE CHICKEN SALAD

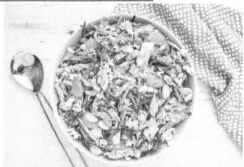

Preparation Time: 15 minutes
Cooking Time: 30 minutes
Servings: 4
Ingredients:

- For the chicken salad:
- 4 divided chicken breasts with skin and bones
- Olive oil of excellent quality
- Salt and freshly ground black pepper
- 500 g asparagus, with the ends removed and cut into three parts diagonally
- 1 red pepper, peeled
- Chinese condiment, recipe to follow
- 2 spring onions (both the white and the green part), sliced diagonally
- 1 tablespoon of white sesame seeds, toasted
- For Chinese dressing:
- 120 ml vegetable oil
- 60 ml of apple cider vinegar of excellent quality
- 60 ml soy sauce
- 1 ½ tablespoon of black sesame
- ½ tablespoon of honey
- 1 clove of garlic, minced
- ½ teaspoon of fresh peeled and grated ginger
- ½ tablespoon sesame seeds, toasted

- 60 g peanut butter
- 2 teaspoons of salt
- ½ teaspoons freshly ground black pepper

Directions:

1. For the chicken salad:
2. Heat the oven to 180°C (or 200°C for gas oven). Put the chicken breast on a baking tray and rub the skin with a little olive oil. Season freely with salt and pepper.
3. Brown for 35 to 40 minutes, until the chicken is freshly cooked. Let it cool down as long as it takes to handle it. Remove the meat from the bones, remove the skin and chop the chicken into medium-sized pieces.
4. Blanch the asparagus in a pot of salted water for 3-5 minutes until tender. Soak them in water with ice to stop cooking. Drain them. Cut the peppers into strips the same size as the asparagus. In a large bowl, mix the chopped chicken, asparagus and peppers.
5. Spread the Chinese dressing on chicken and vegetables. Add the spring onions and sesame seeds, and season to taste. Serve cold or at room temperature.
6. For Chinese dressing:
7. Mix all ingredients and set aside until use.

Nutrition:
Calories 222
Protein 28
Fat 10
Sugar 6

CHICKEN SALAD

Preparation Time: 15 minutes
Cooking Time: 25 minutes
Servings: 4
Ingredients:

- For the Buffalo chicken salad:
- 2 chicken breasts (225 g) peeled, boned, cut in half
- 2 tablespoons of hot cayenne pepper sauce (or another type of hot sauce), plus an addition depending on taste
- 2 tablespoons of olive oil
- 2 romaine lettuce heart, cut into 2 cm strips
- 4 celery stalks, finely sliced
- 2 carrots, roughly grated
- 2 fresh onions, only the green part, sliced
- 125 ml of blue cheese dressing, recipe to follow
- For the seasoning of blue cheese
- 2 tablespoons mayonnaise
- 70 ml of partially skimmed buttermilk
- 70 ml low-fat white yoghurt
- 1 tablespoon of wine vinegar
- ½ teaspoon of sugar
- 35 g of chopped blue cheese
- Salt and freshly ground black pepper

Directions:

1. For the Buffalo chicken salad:
2. Preheat the grid.
3. Place the chicken between 2 sheets of baking paper and beat it with a meat tenderizer so that it is about 2 cm thick, then cut the chicken sideways creating 1 cm strips.
4. In a large bowl, add the hot sauce and oil, add the chicken and turn it over until it is well soaked. Place the chicken on a baking tray and grill until well cooked, about 4-6 minutes, turning it once.

5. In a large bowl, add the lettuce, celery, grated carrots and fresh onions. Add the seasoning of blue cheese. Distribute the vegetables in 4 plates and arrange the chicken on each of the dishes. Serve with hot sauce on the side.
6. For the blue cheese dressing:
7. Cover a small bowl with absorbent paper folded in four. Spread the yoghurt on the paper and put it in the fridge for 20 minutes to drain and firm it.
8. In a medium bowl, beat the buttermilk and firm yogurt with mayonnaise until well blended. Add the vinegar and sugar and keep beating until well blended. Add the blue cheese and season with salt and pepper to taste.

Nutrition:
321 calories
Fat 3
Fiber 5
Carbs 7
Protein 4

TOFU MEAT AND SALAD

Preparation Time: 15 minutes
Cooking Time: 20 minutes
Servings: 3
Ingredients:

- 1 tablespoon of garlic sauce and chili in a bottle
- 1 1/2 tablespoon sesame oil
- 3 tablespoons of low-sodium soy sauce
- 60 ml hoisin sauce
- 2 tablespoons rice vinegar
- 2 tablespoons of sherry or Chinese cooking wine
- 225 g of extra-solid tofu
- 2 teaspoons of rapeseed oil
- 2 tablespoons of finely chopped fresh ginger
- 4 spring onions, with the green part chopped and set aside, in thin slices
- 225 g of minced lean beef (90% or more lean)
- 25 g of diced Chinese water chestnuts
- 1 large head of cappuccino lettuce, with the leaves separated, but without the outer ones
- 1 red pepper, diced

Directions:

- In a bowl, mix together the garlic and chili sauce, sesame oil, soy sauce, hoisin sauce, vinegar and sherry.
- Cut the tofu into 1 cm thick slices and place them on a kitchen towel. Use the cloth to dab the tofu well to remove as much water as possible. Should take a couple of minutes and about three dish towels. Chop the dry tofu well and set aside.
- Heat the oil in a wok or in a very large pan and medium flame. Add the ginger and the white part of the spring onions and cook until the spring onions become translucent and the ginger fragrant, for about 2-3 minutes. Add the beef and tofu and cook, stirring, until the meat becomes dull and freshly cooked, for about 4-5 minutes. Add the sauce set aside. Reduce the flame and simmer slowly, stirring, for another 3-4 minutes. Add the chestnuts and mix well to incorporate.
- Fill each lettuce leaf with stuffing. Serve by decorating with the green part of the spring onions, red pepper and peanuts.

Nutrition:
Calories 122
Fat 2
Protein 66

ASPARAGUS AND PISTACHIOS VINAIGRETTE

Preparation Time: 10 minutes
Cooking Time: 5minutes
Servings: 2
Ingredients:

- Two 455g bunches of large asparagus, without the tip
- 1 tablespoon of olive oil
- Salt and freshly ground black pepper
- 6 tablespoons of sliced pistachios blanched and boiled
- 1 1/2 tablespoon lemon juice
- 1/4 teaspoon of sugar
- 1 1/2 teaspoon lemon zest

Directions:

1. Preheat the oven to 220°C. Put the grill in the top third of the oven. Place the asparagus on a baking tray covered with baking paper. Sprinkle with olive oil and season with a little salt and pepper. Bake for 15 minutes, until soft.
2. Meanwhile, blend 5 tablespoons of almonds, lemon juice, sugar and 6 tablespoons of water for 1 minute until smooth. Taste and regulate salt. Pour the sauce on a plate and put the spinach on the sauce. Decorate with peel and the remaining spoon of pistachios

Nutrition:
Calories 560
Fat 5
Fiber 2
Carbs 3
Protein 9

TURKEY MEATBALLS

Preparation Time: 30 minutes
Cooking Time: 0 minutes
Servings: 4
Ingredients:

- 255g turkey sausage
- 2 tablespoons of extra virgin olive oil
- One can of 425g chickpeas, rinsed and drained...
- 1/2 medium onion, chopped, 2/3 cup
- 2 cloves of garlic, finely chopped
- 1 teaspoon of cumin
- 1/2 cup flour
- 1/2 teaspoon instant yeast for desserts
- Salt and ground black pepper
- 1 cup of Greek yogurt
- 2 tablespoons of lime juice
- 2 radicchio hearts, chopped
- Hot sauce

Directions:

1. Preheat the oven to 200°C.
2. In a processor, blend the chickpeas, onion, garlic, cumin, 1 teaspoon salt and 1/2 teaspoon pepper until all the ingredients are finely chopped. Add the flour, baking powder and blend to make everything mix well. Transfer to a medium bowl and add the sausage, stirring together with your hands. Cover and refrigerate for 30 minutes.

3. Once cold, take the mixture in spoonful, forming 1-inch balls with wet hands. Heat the olive oil in a pan over medium heat. In two groups, put the falafel in the pan and cook until slightly brown, about a minute and a half per side. Transfer to a baking tray and bake in the oven until well cooked, for about 10 minutes.
4. Mix together the yogurt, lime juice, 1/2 teaspoon salt and 1/4 teaspoon pepper. Divide the lettuce into 4 plates, season with some yogurt sauce.

Nutrition:
Calories 189
Fat 5
Protein 77
Sugar 3

CHICKEN, BACON AND AVOCADO CLOUD SANDWICHES

Preparation Time: 10 minutes
Cooking Time: 25 minutes
Servings: 6
Ingredients:
- For cloud bread
- 3 large eggs
- 4 oz. cream cheese
- ½ tablespoon. ground psyllium husk powder
- ½ teaspoon baking powder
- A pinch of salt
- To assemble sandwich
- 6 slices of bacon, cooked and chopped
- 6 slices pepper Jack cheese
- ½ avocado, sliced
- 1 cup cooked chicken breasts, shredded
- 3 tablespoons. mayonnaise

Directions:
1. Preheat your oven to 300 degrees.
2. Prepare a baking sheet by lining it with parchment paper.
3. Separate the egg whites and egg yolks, and place into separate bowls.
4. Whisk the egg whites until very stiff. Set aside.
5. Combined egg yolks and cream cheese.
6. Add the psyllium husk powder and baking powder to the egg yolk mixture. Gently fold in.
7. Add the egg whites into the egg mixture and gently fold in.
8. Dollop the mixture onto the prepared baking sheet to create 12 cloud bread. Use a spatula to spread the circles around to form ½-inch thick pieces gently.
9. Bake for 25 minutes or until the tops are golden brown.
10. Allow the cloud bread to cool completely before serving. Can be refrigerated for up to 3 days of frozen for up to 3 months. If food prepping, place a layer of parchment paper between each bread slice to avoid having them getting stuck together. Simply toast in the oven for 5 minutes when it is time to serve.
11. To assemble sandwiches, place mayonnaise on one side of one cloud bread. Layer with the remaining sandwich ingredients and top with another slice of cloud bread.

Nutrition:
Calories: 333 kcal Carbs: 5g
Fat: 26g Protein: 19.9g

ROASTED LEMON CHICKEN SANDWICH

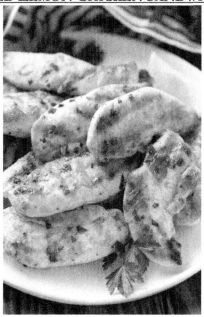

Preparation Time: 15 minutes
Cooking Time: 1 hour 30 minutes
Servings: 12
Ingredients:
- 1 kg whole chicken
- 5 tablespoons. butter
- 1 lemon, cut into wedges
- 1 tablespoon. garlic powder
- Salt and pepper to taste
- 2 tablespoons. mayonnaise
- Keto-friendly bread

Directions:
1. Preheat the oven to 350 degrees F.
2. Grease a deep baking dish with butter.
3. Ensure that the chicken is patted dry and that the gizzards have been removed.
4. Combine the butter, garlic powder, salt and pepper.
5. Rub the entire chicken with it, including in the cavity.
6. Place the lemon and onion inside the chicken and place the chicken in the prepared baking dish.
7. Bake for about 1½ hours, depending on the size of the chicken.
8. Baste the chicken often with the drippings. If the drippings begin to dry, add water. The chicken is done when a thermometer, insert it into the thickest part of the thigh reads 165 degrees F or when the clear juices run when the thickest part of the thigh is pierced.
9. Allow the chicken to cool before slicing.
10. To assemble sandwich, shred some of the breast meat and mix with the mayonnaise. Place the mixture between the two bread slices.
11. To save the chicken, refrigerated for up to 5 days or freeze for up to 1 month.

Nutrition:
Calories: 214 kcal Carbs: 1.6 g
Fat: 11.8 g Protein: 24.4 g.

KETO-FRIENDLY SKILLET PEPPERONI PIZZA

Preparation Time: 10 minutes
Cooking Time: 6 minutes
Servings: 4
Ingredients:
For Crust
½ cup almond flour
½ teaspoon baking powder
8 large egg whites, whisked into stiff peaks
Salt and pepper to taste
Toppings
3 tablespoons. Unsweetened tomato sauce
½ cup shredded cheddar cheese
½ cup pepperoni
Directions
Gently incorporate the almond flour into the egg whites. Ensure that no lumps remain.
Stir in the remaining crust ingredients.
Heat a nonstick skillet over medium heat. Spray with nonstick spray.
Pour the batter into the heated skillet to cover the bottom of the skillet.
Cover the skillet with a lid and cook the pizza crust to cook for about 4 minutes or until bubbles that appear on the top.
Flip the dough and add the toppings, starting with the tomato sauce and ending with the pepperoni
Cook the pizza for 2 more minutes.
Allow the pizza to cool slightly before serving.
Can be stored in the refrigerator for up to 5 days and frozen for up to 1 month.
Nutrition:
Calories: 175 kcal Carbs: 1.9 g Fat: 12 g Protein: 14.3 g.

CHEESY CHICKEN CAULIFLOWER

Preparation Time: 5 minutes
Cooking Time: 10 minutes
Servings: 4
Ingredients:
- 2 cups cauliflower florets, chopped
- ½ cup red bell pepper, chopped
- 1 cup roasted chicken, shredded (Lunch Recipes: Roasted Lemon Chicken Sandwich)
- ¼ cup shredded cheddar cheese
- 1 tablespoon. butter
- 1 tablespoon. sour cream
- Salt and pepper to taste

Directions:
1. Stir fry the cauliflower and peppers in the butter over medium heat until the veggies are tender.
2. Add the chicken and cook until the chicken is warmed through.
3. Add the remaining ingredients and stir until the cheese is melted.
4. Serve warm.

Nutrition:
Calories: 144 kcal Carbs: 4 g Fat: 8.5 g Protein: 13.2 g.

CHICKEN AVOCADO SALAD

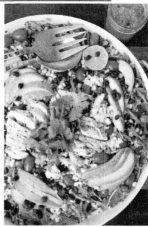

Preparation Time: 7 minutes
Cooking Time: 10 minutes
Servings: 4
Ingredients:
- 1 cup roasted chicken, shredded (Lunch Recipes: Roasted Lemon Chicken Sandwich)
- 1 bacon strip, cooked and chopped
- 1/2 medium avocado, chopped
- ¼ cup cheddar cheese, grated
- 1 hard-boiled egg, chopped
- 1 cup romaine lettuce, chopped
- 1 tablespoon. olive oil
- 1 tablespoon. apple cider vinegar
- Salt and pepper to taste

Directions:
1. Create the dressing by mixing apple cider vinegar, oil, salt and pepper.
2. Combine all the other ingredients in a mixing bowl.
3. Drizzle with the dressing and toss.
4. Can be refrigerated for up to 3 days.

Nutrition:
Calories: 220 kcal
Carbs: 2.8 g
Fat: 16.7 g
Protein: 14.8 g.

CHICKEN BROCCOLI DINNER

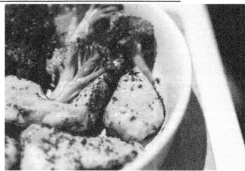

Preparation Time: 10 minutes
Cooking Time: 5 minutes
Servings: 1
Ingredients:
- 1 roasted chicken leg (Lunch Recipes: Roasted Lemon Chicken Sandwich)
- ½ cup broccoli florets

- ½ tablespoon. unsalted butter, softened
- 2 garlic cloves, minced
- Salt and pepper to taste

Directions:

1. Boil the broccoli in lightly salted water for 5 minutes. Drain the water from the pot and keep the broccoli in the pot. Keep the lid on to keep the broccoli warm.
2. Mix all the butter, garlic, salt and pepper in a small bowl to create garlic butter.
3. Place the chicken, broccoli and garlic butter.

Nutrition:

Calories: 257 kcal

Carbs: 5.1 g

Fat: 14 g

Protein: 27.4 g.

EASY MEATBALLS

Preparation Time: 10 minutes

Cooking Time: 20 minutes

Servings: 4

Ingredients:

- 1 lb. ground beef
- 1 egg, beaten
- Salt and pepper to taste
- 1 teaspoon garlic powder
- 1 teaspoon onion powder
- 2 tablespoons. butter
- ¼ cup mayonnaise
- ¼ cup pickled jalapeños
- 1 cup cheddar cheese, grated

Directions

1. Combine the cheese, mayonnaise, pickled jalapenos, salt, pepper, garlic powder and onion powder in a large mixing bowl.
2. Add the beef and egg and combine using clean hands.
3. Form large meatballs. Makes about 12.
4. Fry the meatballs in the butter over medium heat for about 4 minutes on each side or until golden brown.
5. Serve warm with a keto-friendly side.
6. The meatball mixture can also be used to make a meatloaf. Just preheat your oven to 400 degrees F, press the mixture into a loaf pan and bake for about 30 minutes or until the top is golden brown.
7. Can be refrigerated for up to 5 days or frozen for up to 3 months.

Nutrition:

Calories: 454 kcal

Carbs: 5 g

Fat: 28.2 g

Protein: 43.2 g.

CHICKEN CASSEROLE

Preparation Time: 10 minutes

Cooking Time: 40 minutes

Servings: 8

Ingredients:

- 1 lb. boneless chicken breasts, cut into 1" cubes
- 2 tablespoons. butter
- 4 tablespoons. green pesto
- 1 cup heavy whipping cream
- ¼ cup green bell peppers, diced

- 1 cup feta cheese, diced
- 1 garlic clove, minced
- Salt and pepper to taste

Directions

1. Preheat your oven to 400 degrees F.
2. Season the chicken with salt and pepper then batch fry in the butter until golden brown.
3. Place the fried chicken pieces in a baking dish. Add the feta cheese, garlic and bell peppers.
4. Combine the pesto and heavy cream in a bowl. Pour on top of the chicken mixture and spread with a spatula.
5. Bake for 30 minutes or until the casserole is light brown around the edges.
6. Serve warm.
7. Can be refrigerated for up to 5 days and frozen for 2 weeks.

Nutrition:

Calories: 294 kcal

Carbs: 1.7 g

Fat: 22.7 g

Protein: 20.1 g.

LEMON BAKED SALMON

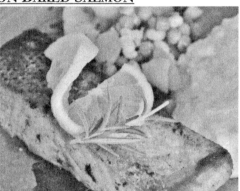

Preparation Time: 10 minutes

Cooking Time: 30 minutes

Servings: 4

Ingredients:

- 1 lb. salmon
- 1 tablespoon. olive oil
- Salt and pepper to taste
- 1 tablespoon. butter
- 1 lemon, thinly sliced
- 1 tablespoon. lemon juice

Directions:

1. Preheat your oven to 400 degrees F.
2. Grease a baking dish with the olive oil and place the salmon skin-side down.
3. Season the salmon with salt and pepper then top with the lemon slices.
4. Slice half the butter and place over the salmon.
5. Bake for 20minutes or until the salmon flakes easily.
6. Melt the remaining butter in a saucepan. When it starts to bubble, remove from heat and allow to cool before adding the lemon juice.
7. Drizzle the lemon butter over the salmon and Serve warm.

Nutrition:

Calories: 211 kcal Carbs: 1.5 g

Fat: 13.5 g Protein: 22.2 g.

CAULIFLOWER MASH

Preparation Time: 10 minutes
Cooking Time: 5 minutes
Servings: 8
Ingredients:

- 4 cups cauliflower florets, chopped
- 1 cup grated parmesan cheese
- 6 tablespoons. butter
- ½ lemon, juice and zest
- Salt and pepper to taste

Directions:

1. Boil the cauliflower in lightly salted water over high heat for 5 minutes or until the florets are tender but still firm.
2. Strain the cauliflower in a colander and add the cauliflower to a food processor
3. Add the remaining ingredients and pulse the mixture to a smooth and creamy consistency
4. Serve with protein like salmon, chicken or meatballs.
5. Can be refrigerated for up to 3 days.

Nutrition:
Calories: 101 kcal
Carbs: 3.1 g
Fat: 9.5 g
Protein: 2.2 g.

ROASTED CHICKEN SOUP

Preparation Time: 10 minutes
Cooking Time: 25 minutes
Servings: 6
Ingredients:

- 4 cups roasted chicken, shredded (Lunch Recipes: Roasted Lemon Chicken Sandwich)
- 2 tablespoons. butter
- 2 celery stalks, chopped
- 1 cup mushrooms, sliced
- 4 cups green cabbage, sliced into strips
- 2 garlic cloves, minced
- 6 cups chicken broth
- 1 carrot, sliced
- Salt and pepper to taste
- 1 tablespoon. garlic powder
- 1 tablespoon. onion powder

Directions:

1. Sauté the celery, mushrooms and garlic in the butter in a pot over medium heat for 4 minutes.
2. Add broth, carrots, garlic powder, onion powder, salt, and pepper.
3. Simmer for 10 minutes or until the vegetables are tender.
4. Add the chicken and cabbage and simmer for another 10 minutes or until the cabbage is tender.
5. Serve warm.
6. Can be refrigerated for up to 3 days or frozen for up to 1 month.

Nutrition:
Calories: 279 kcal
Carbs: 7.5 g
Fat: 12.3 g
Protein: 33.4 g.

CHAPTER 13:

DINNER RECIPES

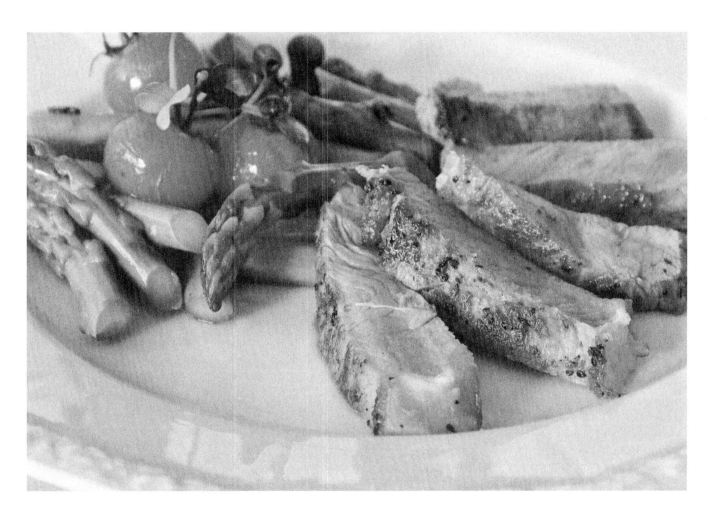

KETO CLOUD BREAD

INGREDIENTS

- Three eggs, separated
- 1/4 teaspoon cream of tartar
- 65g (1/4 cup) crème Fraiche - Pinch salt
- One tablespoon sesame seeds (optional)

METHOD

Preheat oven forced to 150C/130C fan. Bakery paper line two bakery trays.

Using electric beaters in a bowl with an egg whisk attachment and tart cream.

Alternatively, using a fork in a small bowl to whisk the egg yolks, cream fraiche and salt together.

Place the egg yolk mixture with a large metal spoon into the white egg mixture until it is mixed. On the lined tray spoon, two heaped dessertspoonful of the mix. Using the back of a spoon to extend to an 8 cm plate. Repeat to create eight disks with the remaining mixture. If used, sprinkle with sesame seeds.

Bake until golden for 25-30 minutes. Clear slightly from the trays for 10 minutes before switching to a wire rack to cool fully.

LOW-CARB KETO PIZZA DOUGH

INGREDIENTS

- 140g (1 1/3 cups) coarsely grated mozzarella
- 55g (1/2 cup) almond meal
- 2 tablespoons cream cheese
- One egg

METHOD

In a microwave-safe bowl add the grated mozzarella, almond and cream cheese. HIGH microwave (100 percent) for 1 minute, stirring halfway or melted and combined. Add the egg and work hard, beat vigorously until combined with a wooden spoon. Preheat oven forced to 200/180C fan. Place the "dough" between two pieces of bakery paper and put a 32 cm bowl of pizza on a sheet. Remove the top piece of bakery and glue the dough onto the pizza tray with the bottom piece of bakery paper. Prick fork. Prick fork. Bake until golden and puffed for 10 minutes. To slide the pizza out of the tray, use the pad. Switch to the tray to cook from the other side. Cook for another 5 minutes or until the golden end. Complete with your favourite toppings of pizza.

CHEESY SALMON & ASPARAGUS

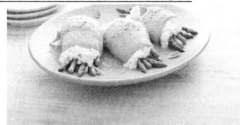

Preparation Time: 15 minutes
Cooking Time: 15 Minutes
Servings: 4

Ingredients:

- 4 Salmon Fillets, 6 Ounces Each & Skin On
- 2 lbs. Asparagus, Trimmed
- 6 Tablespoons Butter
- 4 Cloves Garlic, Minced
- ½ Cup Parmesan Cheese, Grated
- Sea Salt & Black Pepper to Taste

Directions:

1. Start by heating your oven to 400, lining a baking sheet with foil.
2. Pat your salmon dry, seasoning with salt and pepper.
3. Put your salmon in a pan, arranging your asparagus around it.
4. Put a saucepan over medium heat and melt your butter. Add in your garlic, stirring until it browns which takes about three minutes. Drizzle this butter over your salmon and asparagus.
5. Top with parmesan cheese and then cook for twelve minutes. Broil for another three before serving warm.

Nutrition:
Calories: 434 Protein: 42 Grams
Fat: 26 Grams Net Carbs: 6 Grams

HERB PORK CHOPS

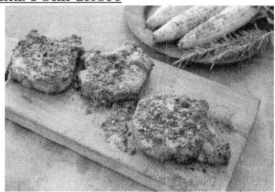

Preparation Time: minutes
Cooking Time: 30 Minutes
Servings: 4
Ingredients:

- 2 Tablespoons Butter + More for Coating
- 4 Pork Chops, Boneless
- 2 Tablespoons Italian Seasoning
- 2 Tablespoons Italian Leaf Parsley Chopped
- 2 Tablespoons Olive Oil
- Sea Salt & Black Pepper to Taste

Directions:

1. Start by heating your oven to 350 and coat a baking dish with butter.
2. Season your pork chops, and then top with fresh parsley, drizzling with olive oil and a half a tablespoon of butter each to bake.
3. Bake for twenty to twenty-five minutes.

Nutrition:
Calories: 333
Protein: 31 Grams
Fat: 23 Grams
Net Carbs: 0 Grams

PAPRIKA CHICKEN

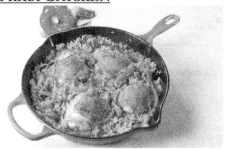

Preparation Time: 15 minutes
Cooking Time: 20 Minutes
Servings: 4
Ingredients:

- 2 Teaspoons Smoked Paprika
- ½ Cup Heavy Whipping Cream
- ½ Cup Sweet Onion, Chopped
- 1 Tablespoon Olive Oil
- 4 Chicken Breasts, Skin On & 4 Ounces Each
- ½ Cup Sour Cream
- 2 Tablespoons Parsley, Chopped

Directions:

1. Season your chicken with salt and pepper, putting a skillet over medium-high heat. Add your oil, and once it simmers, sear your chicken on both sides. It should take about fifteen minutes to cook your chicken all the way through. Put your chicken to the side.
2. Add in your onion, sautéing for four minutes or until tender.
3. Stir in your paprika and cream, bringing it to a simmer.
4. Return your chicken to the skillet, simmering for five more minutes.
5. Stir in sour cream and serve topped with parsley.

Nutrition:
Calories: 389
Protein: 25 Grams
Fat: 30 Grams
Net Carbs: 4 Grams

COCONUT CHICKEN

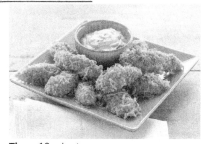

Preparation Time: 10 minutes
Cooking Time: 30 Minutes
Servings: 4
Ingredients:

- 1 Teaspoon Ground Cumin
- 1 Teaspoon Ground Coriander
- ¼ Cup Cilantro, Fresh & Chopped
- 1 Cup Coconut Milk
- 1 Tablespoon Curry Powder

- ½ Cup Sweet Onion, Chopped
- 2 Tablespoons Olive Oil
- 4 Chicken Breasts, 4 Ounces Each & Cut into 2 Inch Chunks

Directions:

1. Get out a saucepan, adding in your oil and heating it over medium-high heat.
2. Sauté your chicken until it's almost completely cooked, which will take roughly ten minutes.
3. Add in your onion, cooking for another three minutes.
4. Whisk your curry powder, coconut milk, coriander and cumin together.
5. Pour the sauce into your pan, bringing it to a boil with your chicken.
6. Reduce the heat, and let it simmer for ten minutes.
7. Serve topped with cilantro.

Nutrition:
Calories: 382
Protein: 23 Grams
Fat: 31 Grams
Net Carbs: 4 Grams

CABBAGE & CHICKEN PLATES

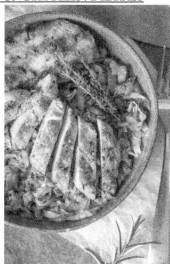

Preparation Time: 25 minutes
Cooking Time: 0 Minutes
Servings: 4
Ingredients:

- 1 Cup Bean Sprouts, Fresh
- 2 Tablespoons Sesame & Garlic Flavored Oil
- ½ Cup Onion, Sliced
- 4 Cups Bok Choy, Shredded
- 3 Stalks Celery, Chopped
- 1 Tablespoon Ginger, Minced
- 2 Tablespoon Coconut Aminos
- 1 Teaspoon Stevia
- 1 Cup Chicken Broth
- 1 ½ Teaspoons Minced Garlic
- 1 Teaspoon Arrowroot
- 4 Chicken Breasts, Boneless, Cooked & Sliced Thin

Directions:

1. Shred your cabbage, and then add your chicken and onion together.

2. Add in a dollop of mayonnaise if desired, drizzling with oil
3. Season as desired and serve.

Nutrition:
Calories: 368 Protein: 42 Grams
Fat: 18 Grams
Net Carbs: 8 Grams

GRILLED CHICKEN & CHEESY SPINACH

Preparation Time: 7minutes
Cooking Time: 6 Minutes
Servings: 6
Ingredients:

- 3 Ounces Mozzarella Cheese, Part Skim
- 3 Chicken Breasts, Large & Sliced in Half
- 10 Ounces Spinach, Frozen, Thawed & Drained
- ½ Cup Roasted Red Peppers, Sliced into Strips
- 2 Cloves Garlic Minced
- 1 Teaspoon Olive Oil
- Sea Salt & Black Pepper to Taste

Directions:

1. Start by heating your oven to 400, and then grease a pan.
2. Bake your chicken breasts for two to three minutes per side.
3. In another skillet, cook your garlic and spinach in oil for three minutes.
4. Put your chicken on a pan, topping it with spinach, roasted peppers and mozzarella.
5. Bake until your cheese melts and serve warm.

Nutrition:
Calories: 195
Protein: 30 Grams
Fat: 7 Grams
Net Carbs: 3 Grams

BALSAMIC CHICKEN WITH VEGETABLES

Preparation Time: 15 minutes
Cooking Time: 25 Minutes
Servings: 4
Ingredients:

- 8 chicken Cutlets, Skinless & Boneless
- ½ Cup Buttermilk, Low Fat
- 4 Tablespoons Dijon Mustard
- 2/3 Cup Almond Meal
- 2/3 Cup Cashews Chopped
- 4 Teaspoons Stevia
- ¾ Teaspoon Rosemary
- Sea Salt & Black Pepper to Taste

Directions:

1. Start by heating your oven to 425.
2. Mix your buttermilk and mustard together in a bowl
3. Add your chicken, coating it.
4. Put a skillet over medium heat, and then add in your almond meal. Bake until its golden, putting it in a bowl.
5. Add your sea salt, pepper, rosemary and cashews, mixing well. Coat your chicken with the almond meal mix, and then put it in a baking pan.
6. Bake for twenty-five minutes.

Nutrition:
Calories: 248
Protein: 27 Grams
Fat: 8 Grams Net
Carbs: 14 Grams

STEAK & BROCCOLI MEDLEY

Preparation Time: 10 minutes
Cooking Time: 10 Minutes
Servings: 4
Ingredients:

- 4 Ounces Butter
- ¾ lb. Ribeye Steak
- 9 Ounces Broccoli
- 1 Yellow Onion
- 1 Tablespoon Coconut Aminos
- 1 Tablespoon Pumpkin Seeds
- Sea Salt & Black Pepper as Needed

Directions:

1. Slice your onion and steak before chopping your broccoli.
2. Put a frying pan over medium heat, adding in butter. Let it melt, and then add meat. Season with salt and pepper, placing your meat to the side.
3. Brown your onion and broccoli, adding more butter as necessary.
4. Add in your coconut aminos before adding your meat back.
5. Serve topped with pumpkin seeds and butter.

Nutrition:
Calories: 875
Protein: 40 Grams
Fat: 75 Grams Net
Carbs: 10 Grams

STUFFED MEAT LOAF

Preparation Time: 20 minutes
Cooking Time: 1 Hour
Servings: 8
Ingredients:

- 17 Ounces Ground Beef
- ¼ Cup Onions, Diced
- 6 Slices Cheddar Cheese
- ¼ Cup Green Onions, Diced
- ½ Cup Spinach
- ¼ Cup Mushrooms

Directions:

1. Mix your salt, pepper, meat, cumin and garlic together before greasing a pan.
2. Put your cheese on the bottom of your meatloaf, adding in the spinach, mushrooms and onions, and then use leftover meat to cover the top.
3. Bake at 350 for an hour before serving.

Nutrition:
Calories: 248
Protein: 15 Grams
Fat: 20 Grams
Net Carbs: 1 Gram

Beef Cabbage Rolls

Preparation Time: 20 minutes
Cooking Time: 6 Hours 10 Minutes
Servings: 5
Ingredients:

- 3 ½ lb. Corned Beef
- 15 Cabbage Leaves, Large
- 1 Onion
- 1 Lemon
- ¼ Cup Coffee
- ¼ Cup White Wine
- 1 Tablespoon Bacon Fat, Rendered
- 1 Tablespoon Brown Mustard
- 2 Tablespoons Himalayan Pink Sea Salt
- 2 Tablespoons Worcestershire Sauce
- 1 Teaspoon Whole Peppercorns
- 1 Teaspoon Mustard Seeds
- ½ Teaspoon Red Pepper Flakes
- ¼ Teaspoons Cloves
- ¼ Teaspoon Allspice
- 1 Bay Leaf, Large

Directions:

1. Add your liquids, corned beef and spices into a slow cooker, cooking on low for six hours.
2. Bring a pot of water to a boil, adding your cabbage leaves and one sliced onion, bringing it to a boil for three minutes.
3. Remove your cabbage, putting it in ice water for three to four minutes, continuing to boil your onion.
4. Dry the leaves off, slicing your meat, and adding in your cooked onion and meat into your leaves.

Nutrition:
Calories: 481 Protein: 35 Grams
Fat: 25 Grams Net Carbs: 4 Grams

Zucchini Fettuccine with Beef

Preparation Time: 15 minutes
Cooking Time: 30 minutes
Servings: 4
Ingredients:

- 15 oz. ground beef
- 3 tbsp butter
- 1 yellow onion
- 8 oz. mushrooms
- 1 tbsp dried thyme
- ½ tsp salt
- 1 pinch ground black pepper
- 8 oz. blue cheese
- 1½ cups sour cream

Zucchini fettuccine:

- 2 zucchinis
- 1 oz. olive oil or butter
- Salt and pepper

Directions:

1. Peel the onion and chop it finely.
2. Melt the butter and sauté the onion until the onions are softened and transparent.

3. Add the ground beef and fry this for a few more minutes with the onion until it is browned and cooked through.
4. Slice or dice the mushrooms, and add it to the ground beef. Sauté the mushrooms with the beef mixture for a few minutes more, or until lightly brown.
5. Season it with thyme, salt, and pepper. Crumble the cheese over the hot mixture. Stir it well.
6. Add the sour cream and bring the mixture to a light boil. Lower the heat to a medium-low setting and let it simmer for about 10 minutes.

Zucchini fettuccine:

1. Calculate about one medium-sized zucchini per person.
2. Slice the zucchini lengthwise in half.
3. Scoop out the seeds with a spoon and slice the halves super thinly, lengthwise (julienne) with a potato peeler, or you can use a spiralizer to make zoodles (zucchini noodles.)
4. Toss the zucchini in some hot sauce of your choice and serve it immediately.
5. If you are not going to be serving your zucchini with a hot sauce, then boil half a gallon of salted water in a large pot and parboil the zucchini slices for a minute. This makes them easier to eat
6. Drain the water from the pot and add some olive oil or a knob of butter. Salt and pepper to taste.

Nutrition:
Calories: 456 Protein: 32 Grams
Fat: 15 Grams Net Carbs: 13 Gram

Oven-Baked Chicken in Garlic Butter

Preparation Time: 25 minutes
Cooking Time: 1 hour 30 minutes
Servings: 3
Ingredients:

- 3 lbs. chickens, a whole bird
- 2 tsp sea salt
- ½ tsp ground black pepper
- 51/3 oz. butter
- 2 garlic cloves, minced

Directions:

1. Preheat the oven to 400°F.
2. Season the chicken with salt and pepper, both inside and out.
3. The chicken must go breast side up in the baking dish.
4. Combine the garlic and butter in a saucepan over a medium heat. The butter should not turn brown or burn, just melt it gently.
5. Let the butter cool down once it is melted.
6. Pour the garlic butter mixture all over and inside the chicken. Bake the chicken on the lower oven rack for 1 to 1 ½ hours, or until internal temperature reaches 180°F. Baste it with the juices from the bottom of the pan every 20 minutes.
7. Serve with the juices.

Nutrition:
Calories: 148
Protein: 39 Grams
Fat: 24 Grams
Net Carbs: 16 Gram

KETO CHICKEN GARAM MASALA

Preparation Time: 10 minutes
Cooking Time: 20 minutes
Servings: 4
Ingredients:

- 25 oz. chicken breasts
- 3 tbsp butter or ghee
- Salt
- 1 red bell pepper, finely diced
- 1¼ cups coconut cream or heavy whipping cream
- 1 tbsp fresh parsley, finely chopped
- Garam masala:
- 1 tsp ground cumin
- 1 - 2 tsp coriander seed, ground
- 1 tsp ground cardamom (green)
- 1 tsp turmeric, ground
- 1 tsp ground ginger
- 1 tsp paprika powder
- 1 tsp chili powder
- 1 pinch ground nutmeg

Directions:

1. Preheat the oven to 400°F.
2. Mix the spices together for the Garam masala.
3. Cut the chicken breasts lengthwise. Place a large skillet over medium-high heat and fry the chicken in the butter until it is golden-brown.
4. Add half of the garam masala spice mix to the pan and stir it thoroughly.
5. Season with some salt, and place the chicken and all of the juices, into a baking dish.
6. Finely chop the bell pepper and add it to a bowl along with the coconut cream and the remaining half of the garam masala spice mix.
7. Pour over the chicken. Bake for 20 minutes.
8. Garnish with parsley and serve.

Nutrition:
Calories: 312 Protein: 21 Grams
Fat: 14 Grams Net Carbs: 2 Gram

KETO LASAGNA

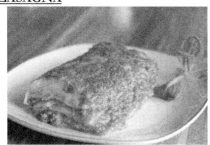

Preparation Time: 25 minutes
Cooking Time: 1 hour minutes
Servings: 4
Ingredients:

- 2 tbsp olive oil
- 1 yellow onion
- 1 garlic clove
- 20 oz. ground beef
- 3 tbsp tomato paste
- ½ tbsp dried basil
- 1 tsp salt
- ¼ tsp ground black pepper
- ½ cup water
- Keto pasta
- 8 eggs
- 10 oz. cream cheese
- 1 tsp salt
- 5 tbsp ground psyllium husk powder

Cheese topping:

- 2 cups crème fraiche or sour cream
- 5 oz. shredded cheese
- 2 oz. grated parmesan cheese
- ½ tsp salt
- ¼ tsp ground black pepper
- ½ cup fresh parsley, finely chopped

Directions:

1. Start with the ground beef mixture.
2. Peel and finely chop the onion and the garlic. Fry them in olive oil until they are soft. Add the ground beef to the onion and garlic and cook until it is golden. Add the tomato paste and remaining spices.
3. Stir the mixture thoroughly and add some water. Bring it to a boil, turn the heat down, and let it simmer for at least 15 minutes, or until the majority of the water has evaporated. The lasagna sheets used don't soak up as much liquid as regular ones, so the mixture should be quite dry.
4. While that is happening, make the lasagna sheets according to the instructions that follow below.
5. Preheat the oven to 400°F. Mix the shredded cheese with sour cream and the Parmesan cheese. Reserve one or two tablespoons of the cheese aside for the topping. Add salt and pepper for taste and stir in the parsley.
6. Place the lasagna sheets and pasta sauce in layers in a greased baking dish.
7. Spread the crème fraiche mixture and the reserved Parmesan cheese on top.
8. Bake the lasagna in the oven for around 30 minutes or until the lasagna has a nicely browned surface. Serve with a green salad and a light dressing.

Lasagna sheets:

1. Preheat the oven to 300°F.
2. Add the eggs, cream cheese, and the salt to a mixing bowl and blend into a smooth batter. Continue to whisk this while adding in the ground psyllium husk powder, just a little bit at a time. Let it sit for a few minutes.
3. Using a spatula spread the batter onto a baking sheet that is lined with parchment paper. Place more parchment paper on top and flatten it with a rolling pin until the mixture is at least 13" x 18". You can also divide it into two separate batches and use a different baking sheet for even thinner pasta.
4. Let the pieces of parchment paper stay in place. Bake the pasta for about 10 to12 minutes. Let it cool and remove the paper. Slice into sheets.

Nutrition:
Calories: 128
Protein: 25 Grams
Fat: 15 Grams
Net Carbs: 4 Gram

KETO BUFFALO DRUMSTICKS AND CHILI AIOLI

Preparation Time: 12 minutes
Cooking Time: 40 minutes
Servings: 6
Ingredients:

- 2 lbs. chicken drumsticks or chicken wings
- 2 tbsp olive oil or coconut oil
- 2 tbsp white wine vinegar
- 1 tbsp tomato paste
- 1 tsp salt
- 1 tsp paprika powder
- 1 tablespoon Tabasco
- Butter or olive oil, for greasing the baking dish

Chili aioli:

- 2/3 cup mayonnaise
- 1 tablespoon smoked paprika powder or smoked chili powder
- 1 garlic clove, minced

Directions:

1. Preheat the oven to 450° (220°C).
2. Put the drumsticks in a plastic bag.
3. Mix the ingredients for the marinade and pour into the plastic bag. Shake the bag and let marinate for 10 minutes.
4. Coat a baking dish with oil. Place the drumsticks in the baking bowl and let bake for 30–40 minutes or until they are done and have turned a beautiful color.
5. Mix together mayonnaise, garlic, and chili.

Nutrition:
Calories: 409
Protein: 22 Grams
Fat: 10 Grams
Net Carbs: 6 Gram

KETO FISH CASSEROLE

Preparation Time: 10 minutes
Cooking Time: 20 minutes
Servings: 4
Ingredients:

- 2 tbsp olive oil
- 15 oz. broccoli
- 6 scallions
- 2 tbsp small capers
- 1/6 oz. butter, for greasing the casserole dish
- 25 oz. white fish, in serving-sized pieces
- 1¼ cups heavy whipping cream
- 1 tbsp Dijon mustard
- 1 tsp salt
- ¼ tsp ground black pepper
- 1 tbsp dried parsley
- 3 oz. butter

Directions:

1. Preheat the oven to 400°F.
2. Divide the broccoli into smaller floret heads and include the stems. Peel it with a sharp knife or a potato peeler if the stem is rough or leafy.
3. Fry the broccoli florets in oil on a medium-high heat for about 5 minutes, until they are golden and soft. Season with salt and pepper to taste.
4. Add finely chopped scallions and the capers. Fry this for another 1 to 2 minutes and place the vegetables in a baking dish that has been greased.
5. Place the fish tightly in amongst the vegetables.
6. Mix the parsley, whipping cream and mustard together. Pour this over the fish and vegetables. Top it with slices of butter.
7. Bake the fish until it is cooked through, and it flakes easily with a fork. Serve as is, or with a tasty green salad.

Nutrition:
Calories: 314
Protein: 20 Grams
Fat: 8 Grams
Net Carbs: 5 Gram

SLOW COOKER KETO PORK ROAST

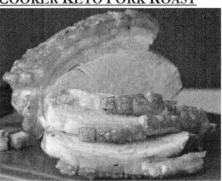

Preparation Time: 35 minutes
Cooking Time: 8 hours 20 minutes
Servings: 4
Ingredients:

- 30 oz. pork shoulder or pork roast
- ½ tbsp salt
- 1 bay leaf
- 5 black pep
- percorns
- 2½ cups water
- 2 tsp dried thyme or dried rosemary
- 2 garlic cloves
- 1½ oz. fresh ginger
- 1 tbsp olive oil or coconut oil
- 1 tbsp paprika powder
- ½ tsp ground black pepper

Creamy gravy:

- 1½ cups heavy whipping cream
- Juices from the roast

Directions:

1. Preheat the oven to a low heat of 200°F.
2. Season the meat with salt and place it into a deep baking dish.
3. Add water. Add a bay leaf, peppercorns, and thyme for more seasoning. Place the baking bowl in the oven for 7 to 8 hours and cover it with aluminum foil.
4. If you are using a slow cooker for this, do the same process as in step 2, only add 1 cup of water. Cook it for 8 hours on low or for 4 hours on high setting.
5. Take the meat out of the baking dish, and reserve the pan juices in a separate pan to make gravy.
6. Turn the oven up to 450°F.

7. Finely chop or press the garlic and ginger into a small bowl. Add the oil, herbs, and pepper and stir well to combine together.
8. Rub the meat with the garlic and herb mixture.
9. Return the meat back to the baking dish, and roast it for about 10 to 15 minutes or until it looks golden-brown.
10. Cut the meat into thin slices to serve it with the creamy gravy and a fibrous vegetable side dish

Gravy:
1. Strain the reserved pan juices to get rid of any solid pieces from the liquid. Boil and reduce the pan juices to about half the original volume, this should be about 1 cup.
2. Pour the reduction into a pot with the whipping cream. Bring this to a boil. Reduce the heat and let it simmer to your desired consistency for a creamy gravy.

Nutrition:
Calories: 432 Protein: 15 Grams
Fat: 29 Grams Net Carbs: 13 Gram

FRIED EGGS WITH KALE AND PORK

Preparation Time: 15 minutes
Cooking Time: 20 minutes
Servings: 5
Ingredients:
- ½ lb. kale
- 3 oz. butter
- 6 oz. smoked pork belly or bacon
- ¼ cup frozen cranberries
- 1 oz. pecans or walnuts
- 4 eggs
- Salt and pepper

Directions:
1. Cut and chop the kale into large squares. You can use pre-washed baby kale as a shortcut if you want. Melt two-thirds of the butter in a frying pan, and fry the kale on high heat until it is slightly browned around its edges.
2. Remove the kale from the frying pan and put it aside. Sear the pork belly in the same frying pan until it is crispy.
3. Turn the heat down. Put the sautéed kale back into the pan and add the cranberries and nuts. Stir this mixture until it is warmed through. Put it into a bowl on the side.
4. Turn up the heat once more, and fry the eggs in the remaining amount of the butter. Add salt and pepper to taste. Serve the eggs and greens immediately.

Nutrition:
Calories: 180 Protein: 23 Grams
Fat: 30 Grams Net Carbs: 13 Gram

CAULIFLOWER SOUP WITH PANCETTA

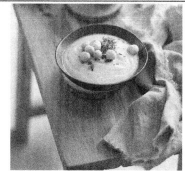

Preparation Time: 15 minutes
Cooking Time: 35 minutes
Servings: 4
Ingredients:
- 4 cups chicken broth or vegetable stock
- 15 oz. cauliflower
- 7 oz. cream cheese
- 1 tbsp Dijon mustard
- 4 oz. butter
- Salt and pepper
- 7 oz. pancetta or bacon, diced
- 1 tbsp butter, for frying
- 1 teaspoon paprika powder or smoked chili powder
- 3 oz. pecans

Directions:
1. Trim the cauliflower and cut it into smaller floret heads. The smaller the florets are, the quicker the soup will be ready.
2. Put aside a handful of the fresh cauliflower and chop into small 1/4 inch bits.
3. Sauté the finely chopped cauliflower and pancetta in butter until it is crispy. Add some nuts and the paprika powder at the end. Set aside the mixture for serving.
4. Boil the cauliflower until they are soft. Add the cream cheese, mustard, and butter.
5. Stir the soup well, using an immersion blender, to get to the desired consistency. The creamier the soup will become the longer you blend. Salt and pepper the soup to taste.
6. Serve soup in bowls, and top it with the fried pancetta mixture.

Nutrition:
Calories: 112
Protein: 10 Grams
Fat: 22 Grams
Net Carbs: 21 Gram

BUTTER MAYONNAISE

Preparation Time: 20 minutes
Cooking Time: 25 minutes
Servings: 4
Ingredients:
- 51/3 oz. butter
- 1 egg yolk
- 1 tbsp Dijon mustard
- 1 tsp lemon juice
- ¼ tsp salt
- 1 pinch ground black pepper

Directions:
1. Melt the butter in a small saucepan. Pour it into a small pitcher or a jug with a spout and let the butter cool.
2. Mix together egg yolks and mustard in a small-sized bowl. Pour the butter in a thin stream while beating it with a hand mixer. Leave the sediment that settles at the bottom.
3. Keep beating the mixture until the mayonnaise turns thick and creamy. Add some lemon juice. Season it with salt and black pepper. Serve this immediately.

Nutrition:
Calories: 428 Protein: 45 Grams
Fat: 4 Grams
Net Carbs: 14 Gram

MEATLOAF WRAPPED IN BACON

Preparation Time: 10 minutes
Cooking Time: 15 minutes
Servings: 3
Ingredients:

- 2 tbsp butter
- 1 yellow onion, finely chopped
- 25 oz. ground beef or ground lamb/pork
- ½ cup heavy whipping cream
- ½ cup shredded cheese
- 1 egg
- 1 tbsp dried oregano or dried basil
- 1 tsp salt
- ½ tsp ground black pepper
- 7 oz. sliced bacon
- 1¼ cups heavy whipping cream, for the gravy

Directions:

1. Preheat the oven to 400°F.
2. Fry the onion until it is soft but not overly browned.
3. Mix the ground meat in a bowl with all the other ingredients, minus the bacon. Mix it well, but avoid overworking it as you do not want the mixture to become dense.
4. Mold the meat into a loaf shape and place it in a baking dish. Wrap the loaf completely in the bacon.
5. Bake the loaf in the middle rack of the oven for about 45 minutes. If you notice that the bacon begins to overcook before the meat is done, cover it with some aluminum foil and lower the heat a bit since you do not want burnt bacon.
6. Save all the juices that have accumulated in the baking dish from the meat and bacon, and use to make the gravy. Mix these juices and the cream in a smaller saucepan for the gravy.
7. Bring it to a boil and lower the heat and let it simmer for 10 to 15 minutes until it has the right consistency and is not lumpy.
8. Serve the meatloaf.
9. Serve with freshly boiled broccoli or some cauliflower with butter, salt, and pepper.

Nutrition:
Calories: 308
Protein: 21 Grams
Fat: 8 Grams
Net Carbs: 19 Gram

KETO SALMON WITH BROCCOLI MASH

Preparation Time: 20 minutes
Cooking Time: 15 minutes
Servings: 5
Ingredients:
Salmon burgers:

- 1½ lbs. salmon
- 1 egg
- ½ yellow onion
- 1 tsp salt
- ½ tsp pepper
- 2 oz. butter, for frying
- Green mash

- 1 lb. broccoli
- 5 oz. butter
- 2 oz. grated parmesan
- Salt and pepper

Lemon butter:

- 4 oz. butter at room temperature
- 2 tablespoons lemon juice
- Salt and pepper to taste

Directions:

1. Preheat the oven to 220° F. Cut the fish into smaller pieces and place them along with the rest of the ingredients for the burger, into a food processor.
2. Blend it for 30 to 45 seconds until you have a rough mixture. Don't mix it too thoroughly as you do not want tough burgers.
3. Shape 6 to 8 burgers and fry them for 4 to 5 minutes on each side on a medium heat in a generous amount of butter. Or even oil if you prefer. Keep them warm in the oven.
4. Trim the broccoli and cut it into smaller florets. You can use the stems as well just peel them and chop it into small pieces.
5. Bring a pot of salted water to a boil and add the broccoli to this. Cook it for a few minutes until it is soft, but not until all the texture is gone. Drain and discard the water used for boiling.
6. Use an immersion blender or even a food processor to mix the broccoli with the butter and the parmesan cheese. Season the broccoli mash to taste with salt and pepper.
7. Make the lemon butter by mixing room temperature butter with lemon juice, salt and pepper into a small bowl using electric beaters.
8. Serve the warm burgers with the side of green broccoli mash and a melting dollop of fresh lemon butter on top of the burger.

Nutrition:
Calories: 156
Protein: 15 Grams
Fat: 11 Grams
Net Carbs: 5 Gram

OVEN BAKED SAUSAGE AND VEGETABLES

Preparation Time: 10 minutes
Cooking Time: 25 minutes
Servings: 2
Ingredients:

- 1 oz. butter, for greasing the baking dish
- 1 small zucchini
- 2 yellow onions
- 3 garlic cloves
- 51/3 oz. tomatoes
- 7 oz. fresh mozzarella
- Sea salt
- Black pepper
- 1 tbsp dried basil
- Olive oil
- 1 lb. sausages in links, in links

For **Servings:**

- 1/2 cup mayonnaise

Directions:
1. Preheat the oven to 400°F. Grease the baking dish with butter.
2. Divide the zucchini into bite-sized pieces. Peel and cut the onion into wedges. Slice or chop the garlic.
3. Place zucchini, onions, garlic, and tomatoes in the baking dish. Dice the cheese and place among the vegetables. Season with salt, pepper and basil.
4. Sprinkle olive oil over the vegetables, and top with sausage.
5. Bake until the sausages are thoroughly cooked and the vegetables are browned.
6. Serve with a dollop of mayonnaise.

Nutrition:
Calories: 176
Protein: 31 Grams
Fat: 12 Grams
Net Carbs: 10 Gram

KETO AVOCADO QUICHE

Preparation Time: 15 minutes
Cooking Time: 10 minutes
Servings: 4
Ingredients:
- Pie crust
- ¾ cup almond flour
- 4 tbsp sesame seeds
- 4 tbsp coconut flour
- 1 tbsp ground psyllium husk powder
- 1 tsp baking powder
- 1 pinch salt
- 3 tbsp olive oil or coconut oil
- 1 egg
- 4 tbsp water

Filling:
- 2 avocados, ripe
- Mayonnaise
- 3 eggs
- 2tbspfinely chopped fresh cilantro
- 1 finely chopped red chili
- Onion powder
- Salt
- ½ cup cream cheese
- 1¼ cups shredded cheese

Directions:
1. Preheat the oven to 350° F. Mix all the ingredients together for the pie dough in a food processor until the dough forms into a ball, this takes a few minutes usually. Use your hands or a fork in the absence of a food processor to knead the dough together.
2. Place a piece of parchment paper to a springform pan, no larger than 12 inches around. The springform pan makes it easier to take the pie out when it is done. Grease the pan and the parchment paper.
3. Using an oiled spatula or oil coated fingers, spread the dough into the pan. Bake the crust for 10 minutes.
4. Split the avocado in half. Remove the peel and pit it, and dice the avocado.
5. Take the seeds out from the chili and chop the chili very finely. Combine the avocado and the chili in a bowl and mix them together with the other ingredients.

6. Pour the mixture into the pie crust and bake it for 35 minutes or until it is a light golden brown. Serve it with a green salad.

Nutrition:
Calories: 323 Protein: 45 Grams
Fat: 18 Grams
Net Carbs: 10 Gram

KETO BERRY MOUSSE

Preparation Time: 10 minutes
Cooking Time: 20 minutes
Servings: 4
Ingredients:
- 2 cups heavy whipping cream
- 3 oz. fresh raspberries, strawberries or even blueberries
- 2 oz. chopped pecans
- ½ lemon the zest
- ¼ tsp vanilla extract

Directions:
1. Pour the cream into a bowl and whip it with a hand mixer until soft peaks form. You can use an old whip too, but this will take some time. Add the lemon zest and vanilla once you are almost done whipping the cream mixture.
2. Combine berries and nuts into the whipped cream and stir it thoroughly.
3. Cover the mousse with plastic wrap and let it sit in the refrigerator for 3 or more hours for a firmer mousse. If your goal is to have a less firm consistency, you can eat the dessert right away.

Nutrition:
Calories: 105 Protein: 33 Grams
Fat: 14 Grams
Net Carbs: 20 Gram

CINNAMON CRUNCH BALLS

Preparation Time: 5 minutes
Cooking Time: 10 minutes
Servings: 1
Ingredients:
- Unsalted butter
- Unsweetened shredded coconut
- Groundgreen cardamom
- Vanilla extract
- Ground cinnamon

Directions:
1. Bring the butter to room temperature.
2. Roast the shredded coconut carefully until they turn a little brown.
3. Mix the butter, half of the coconut and spices.
4. Form into walnut-sized balls. Roll in the rest of the coconut.
5. Store in refrigerator or freezer.

Nutrition:
Calories: 432
Protein: 23 Grams
Fat: 3 Grams
Net Carbs: 5 Gram

KETO CHEESECAKE AND BLUEBERRIES

Preparation Time: 15 minutes
Cooking Time: 60 minutes
Servings: 2
Ingredients:
Crust:

- 1¼ cups almond flour
- 2 oz. butter
- 2 tbsp erythritol
- ½ tsp vanilla extract

Filling:

- 20 oz. cream cheese
- ½ cup heavy whipping cream or crème fraiche
- 2 eggs
- 1 egg yolk
- 1 tsp lemon, zest
- ½ tsp vanilla extract
- 2 oz. fresh blueberries (optional)

Directions:

1. Preheat the oven to 350°F.
2. Butter a 9-inch springform and line the base of it with parchment paper.
3. Next, melt the butter for the crust and heat it until it lets off a nutty scent. This will give the crust an almost toffee-like flavor.
4. Remove it from the heat and add the almond flour, and vanilla. Combine these into firm dough and press the dough into the base of the pan. Bake for about 8 minutes, until the crust turns lightly golden. Set the crust aside and allow it to cool while you prepare the filling.
5. Combine together cream cheese, heavy cream, eggs, lemon zest, and the vanilla. Combine these ingredients well and make sure there are no lumps. Pour this cheese mixture over the crust.
6. Raise the heat of the oven to 400°F and bake for another 15 minutes.
7. Lower the heat to 230°F and bake for another 45-60 minutes.
8. Turn off the heat and let the dessert cool in the oven. Remove it when it has cooled completely and place it in the fridge to rest overnight. Serve it with fresh blueberries.

Nutrition:
Calories: 158
Protein: 5 Grams
Fat: 8 Grams
Net Carbs: 21 Gram

KETO GINGERBREAD CRÈME BRULE

Preparation Time: 15 minutes
Cooking Time: 30 minutes
Servings: 6
Ingredients:

- 1¾ cups heavy whipping cream
- 2 tsp pumpkin pie spice
- 2 tbsp erythritol (an all-natural sweetener)
- ¼ tsp vanilla extract
- 4 egg yolks
- ½ clementine (optional)

Directions:

1. Preheat the oven to 360°F.
2. Crack the eggs to separate them and place the egg whites and the egg yolks in two separate bowls. We will only use egg yolks in this recipe, so save the egg whites for a rainy day.
3. Add some cream to a saucepan and bring it to a boil along with the spices, vanilla extract, and sweetener mixed in.
4. Add the warm cream mixture into the egg yolks. Do this slowly, only adding a little bit at a time, while whisking.
5. Pour it into oven-proof ramekins or small Pyrex bowls that are firmly placed in a larger baking dish with large sides.
6. Add some water to the larger dish with the ramekins in it until it's about halfway up the ramekins. Make sure not to get water in the ramekins though. The water helps the cream cook gently and evenly for a creamy and smooth result.
7. Bake it in the oven for about 30 minutes. Take the ramekins out from the baking dish and let the dessert cool.
8. You can enjoy this dessert either warm or cold, you can also add a clementine segment on top of it.

Nutrition:
Calories: 321
Protein: 14 Grams
Fat: 1 Grams
Net Carbs: 11 Gram

TUSCAN CHICKEN

Preparation Time: 10 minutes
Cooking Time: 30 minutes
Servings: 2
Ingredients:

- 1 lb. boneless and skinless chicken thighs
- 3 tbsps. olive oil
- 6 green onions, chopped
- 1 1/2 cups white wine
- 1 1/2 cups chicken broth
- 1 branch of fresh rosemary
- 1/3 cup black and green olives, pitted and roughly chopped
- Salt and pepper

Directions:

1. In a large skillet, brown the chicken in the oil. Salt lightly (be careful, the olives are already salted) and pepper.
2. Add green onions and continue cooking for about 2 minutes. Add half of the white wine and simmer until evaporated.
3. Add half of the broth, rosemary, and olives. Simmer on low heat until the liquid has reduced by half.
4. Add the remaining wine and broth gradually during cooking as soon as the liquid has reduced by half (see note). Return the chicken a few times during cooking to coat it well in the sauce.
5. Simmer over low heat for about 30 minutes, until the chicken becomes fluffy; check that with a fork and check if the sauce has thickened.
6. Adjust seasoning. Remove the rosemary branch.
7. Divide the chicken thighs between 2 containers
8. Lock the containers and store your dinner in the refrigerator

9. Storage, freeze, thaw and reheat guideline:
10. This Tuscan Chicken can be stored in the refrigerator at 40 °F in a plastic container for about 2 days. When you want to consume your dinner, remove the chicken from the refrigerator and microwave it for about 5 minutes.

Nutrition:
Calories: 505
Fat: 42 g
Carbs: 5.8 g
Protein 26 g
Sugar: 1 g;

STEAK WITH BROCCOLI

Preparation Time: 5 minutes
Cooking Time: 5 minutes
Servings: 3
Ingredients:
- 1/2 small thinly sliced red onion
- 3 tbsp of red wine vinegar
- 1 pinch of kosher salt
- 1 Pinch of freshly ground black pepper
- 5 tbsp of divided extra-virgin olive oil
- 1 and 1/4 lb. of cut skirt steak
- 1 tsp of ground coriander
- 1 thinly sliced small head of broccoli
- 4 c. of Mache
- 1/4 Cup roasted sunflower seeds
- 4 oz., 1/4 cup shaved ricotta

Directions:
1. Combine the vinegar and about 1/2 tsp. salt in a bowl. Then set it aside
2. Meanwhile, press the function sauté of your Instant pot and heat about 1 tbsp. in it; then season the steak with the coriander, the salt, and the pepper.
3. Lock the lid of your Instant Pot
4. Cook for about 5 minutes at a temperature of 365°F
5. Add the broccoli, the Mache, the sunflower seeds, and the remaining 4 tbsps. oil to the onions and toss to combine it.
6. Season the steak with 1 pinch of salt and the pepper.
7. Storage, freeze, thaw and reheat guideline:
8. To store your dinner, divide it between 3 containers; then put the containers in the refrigerator at a temperature of about 40°F. When you are ready to serve your dinner, remove the containers from the refrigerator and microwave it for about 4 minutes

Nutrition:
Calories: 460
Fat: 37.6g
Carbs: 8.5 g
Protein 21.7g
Sugar: 2.3g

INSTANT POT KETOGENIC CHILI

Preparation Time: 5 minutes
Cooking Time: 30 minutes
Servings: 2
Ingredients:
- 1 lb. of ground Beef
- 1 lb. of ground Sausage
- 1 Medium, chopped green Bell Pepper
- 1/2 Medium, chopped yellow onion
- 1 can of 6 oz. of tomato paste
- 2 tbsps. olive oil
- 1 tbsp. avocado oil
- 1 Tbsp of chili Powder
- ½ Tbsp of ground Cumin
- 3 to 4 minced garlic cloves
- 1/3 to ½ cup water
- 1 can of 14.05 diced tomatoes in the tomato Juice

Directions:
1. Preheat your Instant pot by pressing the "Sauté" button
2. Add in the olive oil and avocado oil; then add the ground beef and the sausage to the Instant pot and cook until it becomes brown.
3. Once the meat is browned set the Instant Pot to the function "keep warm/cancel."
4. Add in the rest of the **Ingredients:** into your Instant Pot and mix very well.
5. Cover the lid of the instant pot and lock it; then make sure that the steam valve is sealed
6. Select the function Bean/Chilli setting for around 30 minutes
7. Once the chili is perfectly cooked, the Instant Pot will automatically shift to the function mode "Keep Warm
8. Let the pressure release naturally, or you can rather use the quick release method.
9. Divide the chili between 2 containers; then top with chopped parsley
10. Store the containers in the refrigerator for two days

Nutrition:
Calories: 555
Fat: 46.5g
Carbs: 9.1 g
Protein 24.9g
Sugar: 3g

AHI TUNA BOWL

Preparation Time: 10 minutes
Cooking Time: 5 minutes
Servings: 2
Ingredients:
- 1 lb. of diced ahi tuna, chopped
- 1 tbsp of coconut Aminos
- ½ tsp of sesame oil
- 1/4 cup mayonnaise
- 2 tbsps. cream cheese
- 2 Tbsps. sriracha
- 1 Diced, ripe avocado
- 1/2 cup Kimchi
- ½ Cup chopped green onion
- 1 tbsp. avocado oil
- 1 pinch of sesame seeds

Directions:
1. Add the avocado oil to the bowl; then add the diced tuna.
2. Add the coconut aminos, the cream cheese, the sesame oil, the mayo, the sriracha to the bowl and toss it very well to combine.
3. Add the diced avocado and the kimchi to the bowl and combine it very well.

4. Divide the Kimchi between two containers; then add the greens, the cauliflower rice and the chopped green onion with the sesame seeds
5. Store the containers in the refrigerator for 2 days.

Nutrition:
Calories: 345
Fat: 26.5 g
Carbs: 6.6 g
Protein 19.8 g
Sugar: 1.4g

STUFFED SPINACH AND BEEF BURGERS

Preparation Time: 5 minutes
Cooking Time: 8 minutes
Servings: 2
Ingredients:

- 1 lb. of ground chuck roast
- 1 tsp. salt
- ¾ tsp. ground black pepper
- 2 tbsps. cream cheese
- 1 tbsp. avocado oil
- 1 cup firmly packed fresh spinach
- ½ cup shredded mozzarella cheese (4 to 5 oz.)
- 2 tbsps. grated Parmesan cheese

Directions:

1. In a large bowl, combine the ground beef with the salt, and the pepper.
2. Scoop about 1/3 cup the mixture and with wet hands; shape about 4 patties about ½-inch of thickness. Place the patties in the refrigerator.
3. Place the spinach in a saucepan over medium-high heat.
4. Cover the pan and cook for about 2 minutes, until the spinach becomes wilted.
5. Drain the spinach and let cool; then squeeze the spinach
6. Cut the spinach and put it in a bowl; then stir in the mozzarella cheese, the cream cheese, the avocado oil, and the Parmesan.
7. Scoop ¼ cup the stuffing and shape 4 patties; then cover with the remaining 4 patties
8. Seal both the edges of each burger
9. Cup each of the patties with your hands to make it round
10. Press each of the patties a little bit to make a thick layer Heat your grilling pan over a high heat
11. Grill your burgers for about 6 minutes on each of the two sides.
12. Divide the burgers between 2 containers
13. Store in the refrigerator Serve!

Nutrition:
Calories: 450 Fat: 37 g
Carbs: 7 g Protein 22 g
Sugar: 1.9g

KETOGENIC LOW CARB CLOUD BREAD

Preparation Time: 10 minutes
Cooking Time: 15 minutes
Servings: 3
Ingredients:

- 1 tsp. baking powder
- 1 Cup Philadelphia cheese
- 3 Organic egg

Directions:

1. Separate the whites from the yolks of the three eggs. Place the whites in one bowl and the yolks in the other.
2. Add the cheese at room temperature to the yolks and mix with an electric mixer to obtain a fine paste.
3. Add the baking soda to the egg whites and mix with the mixer.
4. Mix both mixtures gently with a spatula.
5. Preheat the oven to 300°F. Spread small circles of dough on parchment paper
6. , cook for 15 to 20 minutes.
7. Once the cloud bread is cooked, set it aside to cool for about 5 minutes
8. Divide the cloud bread between 3 plastic wraps; then plastic the plastic wraps in two containers
9. Store the containers in the refrigerator for 3 days

Nutrition:
Calories: 200 Fat: 17g
Carbs: 2 g Protein 10g Sugar: 3g

KETOGENIC BRUSCHETTA

Preparation Time: 10 minutes
Cooking Time: 45 minutes
Servings: 3
Ingredients:

- 1 tsp. baking powder
- 1 Cup Philadelphia cheese
- 3 Organic egg
- 1 and ½ cups black olives
- 1 caper
- 24 cherry tomatoes
- oregano
- olive oil
- 1 clove of garlic

Directions:

1. Wash, dry and put the peppers on a baking sheet covered with parchment paper.
2. Bake at 400° F for one hour, turning over on the other side after 30 minutes.
3. Put the roasted peppers in a food bag for 15 minutes.
4. Clean the peppers removing the skin and seeds.
5. Put the peppers on a plate and season with olive oil
6. Wash, dry and halve the cherry tomatoes.
7. Heat a peel and roast the tomatoes on both sides.
8. Toss the slices of Pan Bruschetta so that they are crunchy on the outside.
9. Rub the clove of garlic on the slices of bread.
10. Put the pitted olives in the bowl of a blender and mash them.
11. Coat the slices with olive puree, then cover with peppers cut in fillets, add the tomatoes, some capers, sprinkle with oregano and drizzle with a little olive oil

Nutrition:
Calories: 410 Fat: 35g
Carbs: 7.5 g Protein 16g
Sugar: 1g

CAULIFLOWER PIZZA

Preparation Time: 10 minutes
Cooking Time: 20 minutes
Servings: 2
Ingredients:

- 1 cauliflower
- ½ cup grated mozzarella
- 1 organic egg
- 1 cup white ham
- 1 cup mozzarella
- 4 tbsp of tomato sauce
- ½ cup grated cheese
- 1 tsp. oregano

Directions:

1. Cut the cauliflower head into small florets
2. Grate the cauliflower; the heat it for 4 minutes in the microwave
3. Fluff the cauliflower with a fork
4. Mix the egg and grated cheese with drained cauliflower until you obtain the dough
5. Spread the obtained mixture on a sheet of parchment paper and bake at 400°F until golden brown for about 15 to 20 minutes.
6. Garnish your pizza with olive and capers and
7. It's ready
8. Cut the pizza; then divide the portions between 2 containers and store it in the refrigerator for 2 days

Nutrition:
Calories: 430 Fat: 35.4g Carbs: 7 g
Protein 22.8g Sugar: 3g

CHICKEN PIZZAIOLA

Preparation Time: 10 minutes
Cooking Time: 20 minutes
Servings: 3
Ingredients:

- 3 chicken breasts
- 1 tray with ham
- 1 cup pasta sauce
- 1 and ½ cups grated cheese
- 1 Pinch of salt and pepper
- 2 Tbsps. olive oil

Directions:

1. Preheat the oven to 290 °F
2. Place the 3 chicken breasts on a sheet of parchment paper directly on the plate of your oven.
3. Slice the breasts partially and garnish with sauce, ham, and cheese.
4. Cover with grated cheese, season with salt and pepper and drizzle with oil.
5. Bake in a hot oven for 20 minutes
6. Once ready, divide the 2 chicken breasts between three containers
7. Seal the containers very well and store it in the refrigerator for 3 days

Nutrition:
Calories: 453 Fat: 34.8 g
Carbs: 8.9 g Protein 26g
Sugar: 1.5 g

BEEF STROGANOFF WITH PROTEIN NOODLES

Preparation Time: 14 minutes
Cooking Time: 29 min
Servings: 1
Ingredients:

- 2 oz. Barilla Protein Farfalle Pasta
- ½ cup fresh sliced mushrooms
- 2 Tbls of chopped onion
- 1 T butter
- dash of black pepper
- 6 oz. steak, sliced thinly
- 1 T tomato paste
- ¼ tsp of Dijon mustard
- ½ cup beef broth
- ½ small container plain Greek yogurt

Directions:

1. Cook the pasta in water.
2. Place the butter in a Teflon skillet.
3. Next add in the onions, and mushrooms, cook until onions are shiny and water is gone.
4. Add the beef and brown well.
5. Stir in remaining ingredients except the pasta and yogurt.
6. Cook this until the beef is done, approximately 9 minutes.
7. Drain the pasta.
8. If the sauce is too thin, add 1 tsp low carb flax meal and boil to thicken.
9. Turn back down to low. Then add the yogurt to the sauce.
10. Serve the stroganoff over the pasta.

Nutrition:
Calories: 559
Total Fat: 23g;
Protein: 55g
Total Carbs: 4g
Dietary Fiber: 13g
Sugar: 2g
Sodium: 957mg

BEEFY TOSTADAS

Preparation Time: 4 minute
Cooking Time: 9 minutes
Servings: 2
Ingredients:

- ¼ pound ground sirloin
- ¼ cup onions, minced
- 1 tsp garlic, minced
- 1 T olive oil
- ½ cup chopped green, red, and yellow peppers
- ½ cup cheddar cheese, mild or sharp, hand-shredded
- 2 Tortilla factory low-carb tortillas
- 2 T butter
- 1 c Greek yogurt, plain
- 2 T salsa verde

Directions:

1. Brown the tortillas in the butter. Place on a warm plate.
2. Cook the sirloin, onions, garlic, peppers in the olive oil.

3. Place on the tortillas.
4. Top with the cheese.
5. Add the Greek yogurt.
6. Drizzle with the salsa.

Nutrition:
Calories: 735
Total Fat: 48g
Protein: 66g
Total Carbs: 18g
Dietary Fiber: 8g
Sugar: 0g
Sodium: 708mg

BRATWURST GERMAN DINNER

Preparation Time: 4 minutes
Cooking Time: 19 minutes
Servings:
Ingredients:

- 1 Bratwurst sausage
- ½ cup sliced onion
- ½ cup sauerkraut, this includes the liquid
- 1 tsp olive oil
- Sprinkle of black pepper

Directions:

1. Cook the bratwurst and the onion in the olive oil, in a coated skillet.
2. Remove the bratwurst to a plate.
3. Place the sauerkraut into the skillet and cook 3 min.
4. Add the bratwurst and onion back to warm and mingle the flavors.
5. Sprinkle with black pepper and serve.

Nutrition:
Calories: 332 Total Fat: 26g
Protein: 15g Total Carbs: 8g
Dietary Fiber: 9g Sugar: 4g
Sodium: 1188mg

CAJUN BLACKENED FISH WITH CAULIFLOWER SALAD

Preparation Time: 9 minutes
Cooking Time: 9 minutes
Servings: 1
Ingredients:

- 1 cup chopped cauliflower
- 1 tsp red pepper flakes
- 1 T Italian seasonings
- 1 T garlic, minced
- 6 oz. tilapia
- 1 cup English cucumber, chopped with peel
- 2 T olive oil
- 1 sprig dill, chopped
- 1 Sweetener packet
- 3 T lime juice
- 2 T Cajun blackened seasoning

Directions:

1. Mix the seasonings, except the Cajun blackened seasoning, into one bowl.
2. Add 1 T olive oil.
3. Emulsify or whip.
4. Pour the dressing over the cauliflower and cucumber.

5. Brush the fish with the olive oil on both sides.
6. Pour the other 1 T oil into a coated skillet.
7. Press the Cajun seasoning onto both sides of the fish.
8. Cook the fish in the olive oil 3 minutes per side.
9. Plate and serve.

Nutrition:
Calories: 530
Total Fat: 33.5g
Protein: 32g
Total Carbs: 5.5g
Dietary Fiber: 4g
Sugar: 3g
Sodium: 80mg

CHICKEN PARMESAN OVER PROTEIN PASTA

Preparation Time: 9 minutes
Cooking Time: 14 minutes
Servings: 2
Ingredients:

- 1 dash black pepper
- ½ tsp Italian spice mix
- 8 oz. Protein Plus Spaghetti
- ½ hand-shredded Parmesan
- 1 diced zucchini squash
- 1 ½ cups marinara sauce, any brand
- 24 oz. boneless thin chicken cutlets
- 2 T olive oil
- ½ cup grated Mozzarella cheese
- Water, for boiling the pasta

Directions:

1. Boil the pasta with the zucchini in the water.
2. Mix the Italian spices and ¼ cup Parmesan cheese and place in a shallow dish.
3. Brush the chicken pieces with olive oil and press into spice and cheese to coat.
4. Place in skillet with the oil and cook until done.
5. Add the marinara sauce to the skillet to warm, cover the chicken if you desire.
6. Drain the pasta and zucchini, place on plates.
7. Top the chicken with the mozzarella and remaining Parmesan cheese.
8. Place sauce, chicken, and cheese onto spaghetti and serve.

Nutrition:
Calories: 372 Total Fat: 18g
Protein: 56g Total Carbs: 7 g
Dietary Fiber: 2g
Sugar: 6g
Sodium: 1335mg

CHICKEN CHOW MEIN STIR FRY

Preparation Time: 9 minutes
Cooking Time: 14 minutes
Servings: 4
Ingredients:

- 1/2 cup sliced onion
- 2 T Oil, sesame garlic flavored
- 4 cups shredded Bok-Choy

- 1 c Sugar Snap Peas
- 1 cup fresh bean sprouts
- 3 stalks Celery, chopped
- 1 1/2 tsp minced Garlic
- 1 packet Splenda
- 1 cup Broth, chicken
- 2 T Soy Sauce
- 1 T ginger, freshly minced
- 1 tsp cornstarch
- 4 boneless Chicken Breasts, cooked/sliced thinly

Directions:

1. Place the bok-choy, peas, celery in a skillet with 1 T garlic oil.
2. Stir fry until bok-choy is softened to liking.
3. Add remaining ingredients except the cornstarch.
4. If too thin, stir cornstarch into ½ cup cold water. When smooth pour into skillet.
5. Bring cornstarch and chow mein to a one-minute boil. Turn off the heat source.
6. Stir sauce then for wait 4 minutes to serve, after the chow mein has thickened.

Nutrition:
Calories: 368
Total Fat: 18g
Protein: 42g
Total Carbs: 12g
Dietary Fiber: 16g
Sugar: 6g
Sodium: 746mg

COLORFUL CHICKEN CASSEROLE

Preparation Time: 14 minutes
Cooking Time: 14 minutes
Servings: 6
Ingredients:

- 1 cup broth, chicken
- 3 cups cooked chicken, diced
- 4 cups chopped broccoli
- 1 cup assorted colored bell peppers, chopped
- 1 cup cream
- 4 T sherry
- ¼ c hand-shredded Parmesan cheese
- 1 small size can black olives, sliced, drained
- 2 Tortilla Factory low-carb whole wheat tortillas
- ½ c hand-shredded mozzarella

Directions:

1. Place broccoli and chicken broth into a skillet.
2. Top with lid, bring to a boil, and steam until desired crispness. (4 min)
3. Add the peppers, steam for one minute if you don't want them crisp.
4. Add the chicken and stir to heat.
5. Combine the sherry, cream, parmesan, and olives.
6. Tear the tortillas into bite-sized pieces.
7. Stir into the chicken and broccoli.
8. Pour cream sauce over the chicken, stir.
9. Top with hand-shredded mozzarella.
10. Broil in oven until cheese is melted and golden brown.

Nutrition:
Calories: 412
Total Fat: 30g
Protein: 29
Total Carbs: 10g
Dietary Fiber: 9g
Sugar: 1g
Sodium: 712mg

CHICKEN RELLENO CASSEROLE

Preparation Time: 19 minutes
Cooking Time: 29 minutes
Servings: 6
Ingredients:

- 6 Tortilla Factory low-carb whole wheat tortillas, torn into small pieces
- 1 ½ cups hand-shredded cheese, Mexican
- 1 beaten egg
- 1 cup milk
- 2 cups cooked chicken, shredded
- 1 can Ro-tel
- ½ cup salsa verde

Directions:

1. Grease an 8 x 8 glass baking dish
2. Heat oven to 375 degrees
3. Combine everything together, but reserve ½ cup of the cheese
4. Bake it for 29 minutes
5. Take it out of oven and add ½ cup cheese
6. Broil for about 2 minutes to melt the cheese

Nutrition:
Calories: 265
Total Fat: 16g
Protein: 20g
Total Carbs: 18g
Dietary Fiber: 10g
Sugar: 0g
Sodium: 708mg

CHAPTER 14:

SOUP AND STEW

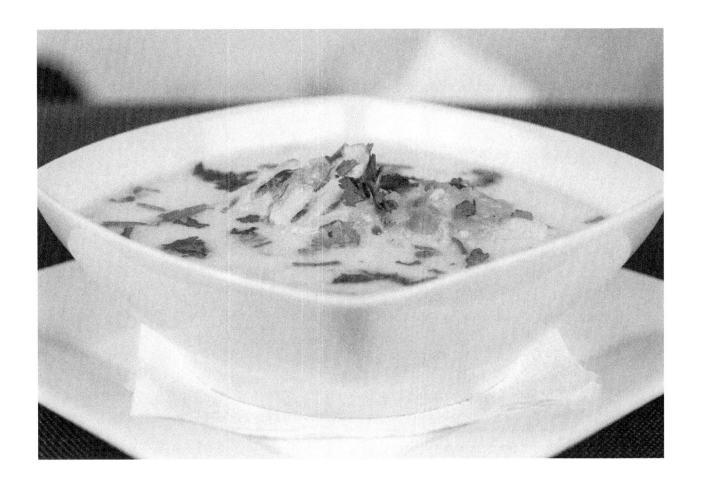

CREAM OF MUSHROOM SOUP WITH TARRAGON OIL

INGREDIENTS

- 40g butter
- One brown onion, roughly chopped
- One garlic clove, crushed
- 200g button mushrooms, chopped
- 200g Swiss brown mushrooms, chopped
- Two medium cream delight potatoes, peeled, roughly chopped
- 3 cups Massel chicken style liquid stock
- 1/4 cup fresh tarragon leaves, plus extra chopped leaves to serve
- 1/4 cup extra virgin olive oil
- 3/4 cup pure cream
- 50g button mushrooms, sliced, extra
- 50g swiss brown mushrooms, sliced, extra

METHOD

In a saucepan, melt 1/2 butter over medium heat. Fill in onion and garlic. Cook, stirring, cook 5 minutes or soft onion. Add champignons. Cook, stirring, 2 to 3 minutes, or tender mushrooms. Stir in carrots, stock and 1 cup of tea. Cover. Cover. Bring to boil. Bring to boil. Reduce to the low sun. Simmer for 20 minutes, wrapped, or tender potato. Set aside to cool slightly for 10 minutes. In the meantime, place the leaves of tarragon and the oil in a small jug. Using a mixer to mix almost smoothly. Move the mixture over a small bowl by a fine sieve. Reject solids. Use a stick blender to mix soup easily. Add milk. Add butter. High heat spot. Low heat spot. Remove for 5 minutes or until warm. Salt and pepper season. Pack. In the meantime, in a frying pot heat remaining butter over medium to high heat. Connect additional mushrooms. Cook for 5 minutes, occasionally stirring, or until golden.

Ladle soup in cups. Top with fried champagne and extra chopped tarragon. Drizzle with olive oil. Honour. Honor.

CHEESY CAULIFLOWER SOUP

Preparation Time: 10 minutes
Cooking Time: 30 minutes
Servings: 8
Ingredients:

- ¼ cup butter
- 1 head cauliflower, chopped
- ½ onion, chopped
- ½ teaspoon ground nutmeg
- 4 cups chicken stock
- 1 cup heavy whipping cream
- Salt and freshly ground black pepper, to taste
- 1 cup Cheddar cheese, shredded

Directions:
1. Take a large stockpot and place it over medium heat.
2. Add butter to this pot and let it melt.
3. Add cauliflower and onion to the melted butter and sauté for 10 minutes until these veggies are soft.
4. Add nutmeg and chicken stock to the pot and bring to a boil.

5. Reduce the heat to low and allow it to simmer for 15 minutes.
6. Remove the stockpot from the heat and then add heavy cream.
7. Purée the cooked soup with an immersion blender until smooth.
8. Sprinkle this soup with salt and black pepper.
9. Garnish with Cheddar cheese and serve warm.

Nutrition:
Calories: 224 Fat: 16.8g
Total carbs: 10.8g Fiber: 2.2g
Protein: 9.6g

EGG BROTH

Preparation Time: 5 minutes
Cooking Time: 5 minutes
Servings: 4
Ingredients:

- 2 tablespoons unsalted butter
- 4 cups chicken broth
- 3 large eggs
- Salt and black pepper, to taste
- 1 sliced green onion, for garnish

Directions:
1. Take a medium stockpot and place it over high heat.
2. Add butter and chicken broth to the pot and bring to a boil.
3. Break eggs into a bowl and beat them for 1 minute with a fork until frothy.
4. Once the broth boils, slowly pour in beaten eggs while stirring the broth with a spoon.
5. Cook for 1 minute with continuously stirring, then sprinkle salt and black pepper to season.
6. Garnish with sliced green onion, then serve warm.

Nutrition:
Calories: 93 Fat: 7.8g
Total carbs: 1.8g Fiber: 0.1g
Protein: 3.9g

CAULIFLOWER CREAM SOUP

Preparation Time: 15 minutes
Cooking Time: 4 hours 10 minutes
Servings: 5
Ingredients:

- 10 slices bacon
- 3 small heads cauliflower, cored and cut into florets
- 4 cups chicken broth
- ¼ cup (½ stick) salted butter
- 3 cloves garlic, pressed
- ½ large yellow onion, chopped
- 1 cup heavy whipping cream
- 2 cups Cheddar cheese, shredded
- Salt and black pepper, to taste
- Freshly chopped chives or green onions, for garnish

Directions:
1. Take a large skillet and place it over medium heat.
2. Add bacon to the skillet and cook for about 8 minutes until brown and crispy.
3. Transfer the cooked bacon to a paper towel-lined plate to absorb the excess grease.
4. Allow the bacon to cool, then chop it. Wrap the plate of chopped bacon in plastic and refrigerate it.

5. Add the cauliflower florets to the food processor and pulse until chopped thoroughly.
6. Add chicken broth, butter, garlic, onion, and chopped cauliflower to the slow cooker.
7. Give all these ingredients a gentle stir, then put on the lid.
8. Cook the cauliflower soup for 4 hours on high heat.
9. Once the cauliflower is tender, purée the soup with an immersion blender until smooth.
10. Add chopped bacon, heavy cream, cheese, salt, and black pepper. Mix well and let the cheese melt in the hot soup.
11. Garnish with green onions or chives, then serve warm.

Nutrition:
Calories: 627
Fat: 54.3g
Total carbs: 13.7g
Fiber: 3.7g
Protein: 24.6g

SHRIMP MUSHROOM CHOWDER

Preparation Time: 10 minutes
Cooking Time: 40 minutes
Servings: 6
Ingredients:

- ¼ cup refined avocado oil
- 1/3 cup diced yellow onions
- 1 2/3 cups diced mushrooms
- 10½ ounces (298 g) small raw shrimp, shelled and deveined
- 1 can (131/2-ounce / 383-g) unsweetened coconut milk
- 1/3 cup chicken bone broth
- 2 tablespoons apple cider vinegar
- 1 teaspoon onion powder
- 1 teaspoon paprika
- 1 bay leaf
- ¾ teaspoon finely ground gray sea salt
- ½ teaspoon dried oregano leaves
- ¼ teaspoon ground black pepper
- 1 medium zucchini (7-ounce / 198-g), cubed
- 12 radishes (6-ounce / 170-g), cubed

Directions:
1. Add avocado oil to a large saucepan and place it over medium heat.
2. Add onions and mushrooms to the pan and sauté for 10 minutes or until onions are soft and mushrooms are lightly browned.
3. Stir in shrimp, coconut milk, chicken broth, apple cider vinegar, onion powder, paprika, bay leaf, sea salt, oregano leaves, and black pepper.
4. Cover the soup mixture with a lid and cook for 20 minutes on low heat.
5. Add zucchini and radishes to the soup and cook for 10 minutes.
6. Remove the bay leaf from the soup and divide the soup into 6 small serving bowls. Serve hot.

Nutrition:
Calories: 311 Fat: 26.3g
Total carbs: 7.7g Fiber: 2.9g
Protein: 13.7g

PORK TARRAGON SOUP

Preparation Time: 10 minutes
Cooking Time: 1 hour 20 minutes
Servings: 6
Ingredients:

- 1/3 cup lard
- 1 pound (454 g) pork loin, cut into ½-inch (1.25-cm) pieces
- 10 strips bacon (about 10-ounce / 284-g), cut into ½-inch (1.25-cm) pieces
- ¾ cup sliced shallots
- 3 medium turnips (about 12½-ounce / 354-g), cubed
- 1 tablespoon yellow mustard
- ¼ cup dry white wine
- 1¾ cups chicken bone broth
- 4 sprigs fresh thyme
- 2 tablespoons unflavored gelatin
- 2 tablespoons apple cider vinegar
- ½ cup unsweetened coconut milk
- 1 tablespoon dried tarragon leaves

Directions:
1. Take a large saucepan and place it over medium heat.
2. Add lard to the saucepan and allow it to melt.
3. Add pork pieces to the melted lard and sauté for 8 minutes until golden brown.
4. Add bacon pieces and sliced shallots and sauté for 5 minutes or until fragrant.
5. Add turnips, mustard, wine, bone broth, and thyme sprigs to the soup.
6. Mix these ingredients gently and cover this soup with a lid.
7. Bring the soup to a boil, then reduce the heat to medium-low. Cook this soup for 1 hour.
8. Remove and discard the thyme sprigs from the soup then add gelatin, vinegar, coconut milk, and tarragon.
9. Increase the heat to medium and bring the soup to a boil. Cover to cook for 10 minutes.
10. Divide the cooked soup into 6 serving bowls and serve warm.

Nutrition:
Calories: 566 Fat: 41.5g
Total carbs: 9.7g Fiber: 1.2g Protein: 39.6g

CREAMY BROCCOLI AND CAULIFLOWER SOUP

Preparation Time: 20 minutes
Cooking Time: 15 minutes
Servings: 6
Ingredients:

- 1 (13½-ounce / 383-g) can unsweetened coconut milk
- 2 cups vegetable stock
- 1 (14-ounce / 397-g) small head cauliflower, cored and cut into large florets
- 2 medium celery sticks, chopped
- 1 teaspoon finely ground gray sea salt
- 6 green onions, green parts only, roughly chopped
- 1 large head broccoli, cored and cut into large florets
- ¼ teaspoon ground black pepper
- ¼ teaspoon ground white pepper
- 1/3 cup butter-infused olive oil
- 1 chopped green onion, for garnish

Directions:

1.   Take a large saucepan and place it over medium heat.
2.   Add coconut milk, vegetable stock, cauliflower florets, chopped celery, salt, and green onions.
3.   Mix them gently, then cover and bring the soup to a boil.
4.   Continue cooking the soup for 15 minutes until the cauliflower florets are soft.
5.   Meanwhile, blanch the broccoli in a pot of boiling water for 1 minute until soft but still crisp, then drain on a paper towel. Set aside on a plate.
6.   When the cauliflower soup is cooked, transfer it to a blender.
7.   Add black pepper, white pepper, and olive oil. Blend the soup for 1 minute until smooth.
8.   Add the soft broccoli and blend again for 30 seconds.
9.   Divide the cooked broccoli and cauliflower soup into 6 serving bowls.
10. Garnish with chopped green onions and serve warm.

Nutrition:
Calories: 264 Fat: 23.3g
Total carbs: 10.3g Fiber: 3.6g
Protein: 6.9g

CHICKEN TURNIP SOUP

Preparation Time: 10 minutes
Cooking Time: 6 to 8 hours
Servings: 5
Ingredients:

- 12 ounces (340g) bone-in chicken
- ¼ cup turnip, chopped
- ¼ cup onions, chopped
- 4 garlic cloves, smashed
- 4 cups water
- 3 sprigs thyme
- 2 bay leaves
- Salt, to taste
- ¼ teaspoon freshly ground black pepper

Directions:

1.   Put the chicken, turnip, onions, garlic, water, thyme springs, and bay leaves in a slow cooker.
2.   Season with salt and pepper, then give the mixture a good stir.
3.   Cover and cook on low for 6 to 8 hours until the chicken is cooked through.
4.   When ready, remove the bay leaves and shred the chicken with a fork.
5.   Divide the soup among five bowls and serve.

Nutrition:
Calories: 186 Fat: 13.6g
Total carbs: 3.3g Fiber: 2.6g
Protein: 15.2g

SPINACH MUSHROOM SOUP

Preparation Time: 10 minutes
Cooking Time: 5 minutes
Servings: 3
Ingredients:

- 1 tablespoon olive oil
- 1 teaspoon garlic, finely chopped
- 1 cup spinach, torn into small pieces
- ½ cup mushrooms, chopped

- Salt and freshly ground black pepper, to taste
- ½ teaspoon tamari
- 3 cups vegetable stock
- 1 teaspoon sesame seeds, roasted

Directions:

1.   Place a saucepan over medium heat and add olive oil to heat.
2.   Add garlic to the hot oil and sauté for 30 seconds or until fragrant.
3.   Add spinach and mushrooms, then sauté for 1 minute or until lightly tender.
4.   Add salt, black pepper, tamari, and vegetable stock. Cook for another 3 minutes. Stir constantly.
5.   Garnish with sesame seeds and serve warm.

Nutrition:
Calories: 80 Fat: 7.4g Total carbs: 3.2g
Fiber: 1.1g Protein: 1.2g

GARLICKY CHICKEN SOUP

Preparation Time: 10 minutes
Cooking Time: 10 minutes
Servings: 4
Ingredients:

- 2 tablespoons butter
- 1 large chicken breast cut into strips
- 4 ounces (113 g) cream cheese, cubed
- 2 tablespoons Garlic Gusto Seasoning
- ½ cup heavy cream
- 14½ ounces (411 g) chicken broth
- Salt, to taste

Directions:

1.   Place a saucepan over medium heat and add butter to melt.
2.   Add chicken strips and sauté for 2 minutes.
3.   Add cream cheese and seasoning, and cook for 3 minutes, stirring occasionally.
4.   Pour in the heavy cream and chicken broth. Bring the soup to a boil, then lower the heat.
5.   Allow the soup to simmer for 4 minutes, then sprinkle with salt.
6.   Let cool for 5 minutes and serve while warm.

Nutrition:
Calories: 243
Fat: 22.5g
Total carbs: 7.0g
Fiber: 6.6g
Protein: 9.6g

CAULIFLOWER CURRY SOUP

Preparation Time: 15 minutes
Cooking Time: 26 minutes
Servings: 4
Ingredients:

- 2 tablespoons avocado oil
- 1 white onion, chopped
- 4 garlic cloves, chopped
- ½ Serrano pepper, seeds removed and chopped
- 1-inch ginger, chopped
- ¼ teaspoon turmeric powder
- 2 teaspoons curry powder
- ½ teaspoon black pepper
- 1 teaspoon salt
- 1 cup of water

- 1 large cauliflower, cut into florets
- 1 cup chicken broth
- 1 can unsweetened coconut milk
- Cilantro, for garnish

Directions:

1. Place a saucepan over medium heat and add oil to heat.
2. Add onions to the hot oil and sauté them for 3 minutes.
3. Add garlic, Serrano pepper, and ginger, then sauté for 2 minutes.
4. Add turmeric, curry powder, black pepper, and salt. Cook for 1 minute after a gentle stir.
5. Pour water into the pan, then add cauliflower.
6. Cover this soup with a lid and cook for 10 minutes. Stir constantly.
7. Remove the soup from the heat and allow it to cool at room temperature.
8. Transfer this soup to a blender and purée the soup until smooth.
9. Return the soup to the saucepan and add broth and coconut milk. Cook for 10 minutes more and stir frequently.
10. Divide the soup into four bowls and sprinkle the cilantro on top for garnish before serving.

Nutrition:
Calories: 342
Fat: 29.1g
Total carbs: 18.3g
Fiber: 5.5g
Protein: 7.17g

Asparagus Cream Soup

Preparation Time: 15 minutes
Cooking Time: 22 minutes
Servings: 6
Ingredients:

- 4 tablespoons butter
- 1 small onion, chopped
- 6 cups low-sodium chicken broth
- Salt and black pepper, to taste
- 2 pounds (907g) asparagus, cut in half
- ½ cup sour cream

Directions:

1. Place a large pot over low heat and add butter to melt.
2. Add onion to the melted butter and sauté for 2 minutes or until soft.
3. Add chicken broth, salt, black pepper, and asparagus.
4. Bring the soup to a boil, then cover the lid and cook for 20 minutes.
5. Remove the pot from the heat and allow it to cool for 5 minutes.
6. Transfer the soup to a blender and blend until smooth.
7. Add sour cream and pulse again to mix well.
8. Serve fresh and warm.

Nutrition:
Calories: 138
Fat: 10.5g
Total carbs: 10.2g
Fiber: 3.5g
Protein: 5.9g

Red Gazpacho Cream Soup

Preparation Time: 15 minutes
Cooking Time: 20 minutes

Servings: 10
Ingredients:

- 1 large red bell pepper, halved
- 1 large green bell pepper, halved
- 2 tablespoons basil, freshly chopped
- 4 medium tomatoes
- 1 small red onion
- 1 large cucumber, diced
- 2 medium spring onions, diced
- 2 tablespoons apple cider vinegar
- 2 garlic cloves
- 2 tablespoons fresh lemon juice
- 1 cup extra virgin olive oil
- Salt and black pepper, to taste
- 1¼ pounds (567 g) feta cheese, shredded

Directions:

1. Preheat the oven to 400°F (205°C) and line a baking tray with parchment paper.
2. Place all the bell peppers in the baking tray and roast in the preheated oven for 20 minutes.
3. Remove the bell peppers from the oven. Allow to cool, then peel off their skin.
4. Transfer the peeled bell peppers to a blender along with basil, tomatoes, red onions, cucumber, spring onions, vinegar, garlic, lemon juice, olive oil, black pepper, and salt. Blend until the mixture smooth.
5. Add black pepper and salt to taste.
6. Garnish with feta cheese and serve warm.

Nutrition:
Calories: 248 Fat: 21.6g Total carbs: 8.3g
Fiber: 4.1g Protein: 9.3g

Beef Taco Soup

Preparation Time: 15 minutes
Cooking Time: 24 minutes
Servings: 8
Ingredients:

- 2 garlic cloves, minced
- ½ cup onions, chopped
- 1 pound (454 g) ground beef
- 1 teaspoon chili powder
- 1 tablespoon ground cumin
- 1 (8-ounce / 227-g) package cream cheese, softened
- 2 (10-ounce / 284-g) cans diced tomatoes and green chilies
- ½ cup heavy cream
- 2 teaspoons salt
- 2 (14½-ounce / 411-g) cans beef broth

Directions:

1. Take a large saucepan and place it over medium-high heat.
2. Add garlic, onions, and ground beef to the soup and sauté for 7 minutes until beef is browned.
3. Add chili powder and cumin, then cook for 2 minutes.
4. Add cream cheese and cook for 5 minutes while mashing the cream cheese into the beef with a spoon.
5. Add diced tomatoes and green chilies, heavy cream, salt and broth then cook for 10 minutes.
6. Mix gently and serve warm.

Nutrition:
Calories: 205 Fat: 13.3g
Total carbs: 4.4g Fiber: 0.8g Protein: 8.0g

CREAMY TOMATO SOUP

Preparation Time: 15 minutes
Cooking Time: 30 minutes
Servings: 4
Ingredients:

- 2 cups of water
- 4 cups tomato juice
- 3 tomatoes, peeled, seeded and diced
- 14 leaves fresh basil
- 2 tablespoons butter
- 1 cup heavy whipping cream
- Salt and black pepper, to taste

Directions:

1. Take a suitable cooking pot and place it over medium heat.
2. Add water, tomato juice, and tomatoes, then simmer for 30 minutes.
3. Transfer the soup to a blender, then add basil leaves.
4. Press the pulse button and blend the soup until smooth.
5. Return this tomato soup to the cooking pot and place it over medium heat.
6. Add butter, heavy cream, salt, and black pepper. Cook and mix until the butter melts.
7. Serve warm and fresh.

Nutrition:
Calories: 203
Fat: 17.7g
Total carbs: 13.0g
Fiber: 5.6g
Protein: 3.7g

CREAMY BROCCOLI AND LEEK SOUP

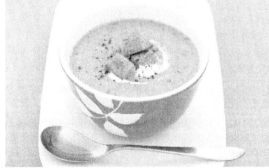

Preparation Time: 5 minutes
Cooking Time: 25 minutes
Servings: 4
Ingredients: 10 oz. broccoli

- 1 leek
- 8 oz. cream cheese
- 3 oz. butter
- 3 cups water
- 1 garlic clove
- ½ cup fresh basil
- salt and pepper

Directions:

1. Rinse the leek and chop both parts finely. Slice the broccoli thinly.
2. Place the veggies in a pot and cover with water and then season them. Boil the water until the broccoli softens.

3. Add the florets and garlic, while lowering the heat.
4. Add in the cheese, butter, pepper, and basil. Blend until desired consistency: if too thick use water; if you want to make it thicker, use a little bit of heavy cream.

Nutrition:
Calories: 451 kcal Fats: 37 g Protein: 10 g
Carbs: 4 g

CHICKEN SOUP

Preparation Time: 25 minutes
Cooking Time: 80 minutes
Servings: 4
Ingredients:

- 6 cups water
- 1 chicken
- 1 medium carrot
- 1 yellow onion
- 1 bay leaf
- 1 leek
- 2 garlic cloves
- 1 tbsp. dried thyme
- ½ cup white wine, dry (no, not for drinking)
- 1 tsp. peppercorns
- salt and pepper

Directions:

1. Peel and cut your veggies. Brown them in oil in a big pot.
2. Split your chicken in half, down on the middle. Pour water and spices in the pot. Let it simmer for one hour.
3. Take out the chicken save the meat, and toss away the bones.
4. Put the meat back in the pot, and let it simmer on medium heat for 20-25 minutes again, while seasoning to your liking.

Nutrition:
Calories: 145 kcal
Fats: 12 g
Carbs: 1 g
Protein: 8 g

GREEK EGG AND LEMON SOUP WITH CHICKEN

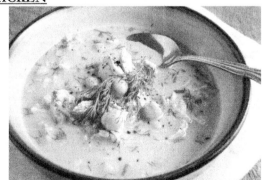

Preparation Time: 5 minutes
Cooking Time: 30 minutes
Servings: 4
Ingredients:

- 4 cups water

- ¾ lbs. cauli
- 1 lb. boneless chicken thighs
- 1/3 lb. butter
- 4 eggs
- 1 lemon
- 2 tbsps. fresh parsley
- 1 bay leaf
- 2 chicken bouillon cubes
- salt and pepper

Directions:

1. Slice your chicken thinly and then place in a saucepan while adding cold water and the cubes and bay leaf. Let the meat simmer for 10 minutes before removing it and the bay leaf.
2. Grate your cauli and place it in a saucepan. Add butter and boil for a few minutes.
3. Beat your eggs and lemon juice in a bowl, while seasoning it.
4. Reduce the heat a bit and add the eggs, stirring continuously. Let simmer but don't boil.
5. Return the chicken.

Nutrition:
Calories: 582 kcal
Carbs: 4 g
Fats: 49 g
Protein: 31 g

WILD MUSHROOM SOUP

Preparation Time: 10 minutes
Cooking Time: 30 minutes
Servings: 4
Ingredients:

- 6 oz. mix of portabella mushrooms, oyster mushrooms, and shiitake mushrooms
- 3 cups water
- 1 garlic clove
- 1 shallot
- 4 oz. butter
- 1 chicken bouillon cube
- ½ lb. celery root
- 1 tbsp. white wine vinegar
- 1 cup heavy whipping cream
- fresh parsley

Directions:

1. Clean, trim, and chop your mushrooms and celery. Do the same to your shallot and garlic.
2. Sauté your chopped veggies in butter over medium heat in a saucepan.
3. Add thyme, vinegar, chicken bouillon cube, and water as you bring to boil. Then let it simmer for 10-15 minutes.
4. Add cream to them with an immersion blender until your desired consistency. Serve with parsley on top.

Nutrition:
Calories: 481 kcal
Fats: 47 g
Protein: 7 g
Carbs: 9 g

ROASTED BUTTERNUT SQUASH SOUP

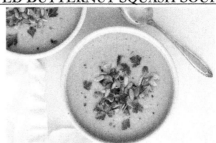

Preparation Time: 15 minutes
Cooking Time: 30 minutes
Servings: 4
Ingredients:

- 1 large butternut squash, cubed and peeled
- 1 stalk celery, sliced
- 2 potatoes, peeled, chopped
- 1 onion, chopped
- 1 large carrot, chopped
- 3 tbsps. olive oil
- 1 tbsp. fresh thyme
- 25 oz. chicken broth
- 1 tbsp. butter
- salt and pepper

Directions:

1. Preheat your oven to 400°F. On a baking sheet, toss squash and potatoes with 2 tbsp. oil and season to your taster. Roast for 20-25 minutes.
2. In the meantime, melt your butter and the rest of the oil in a large pot over medium heat. Add the onion, celery, carrot and cook for 5-8 minutes. Season them, too.
3. Add roasted squash and potatoes. Then pour over the chicken broth. Simmer it for 10 minutes using an immersion blender until the soup is creamy.
4. Garnish it with thyme.

Nutrition:
Calories: 254 kcal
Fats: 15 g
Carbs: 19 g
Protein: 6 g

ZUCCHINI CREAM SOUP

Preparation Time: 5 minutes
Cooking Time: 20 minutes
Servings: 4
Ingredients:

- 3 zucchinis
- 32 oz. chicken broth
- 2 cloves garlic
- 2 tbsps. sour cream
- ½ small onion
- parmesan cheese (for topping if desired)

Directions:

1. Combine your broth, garlic, zucchini, and onion in a large pot over medium heat until boiling.
2. Lower the heat, cover, and let simmer for 15-20 minutes

3. Remove from heat and purée with an immersion blender, while adding the sour cream and pureeing until smooth.
4. Season to taste and top with your cheese.

Nutrition:
Calories: 117 kcal
Fats: 9 g
Carbs: 3 g
Protein: 4 g

CAULI SOUP

Preparation Time: 5 minutes
Cooking Time: 25 minutes
Servings: 6
Ingredients:

- 32 oz. vegetable broth
- 1 head cauli, diced
- 2 garlic cloves, minced
- 1 onion, diced
- ½ tbsp. olive oil
- salt and pepper
- grated parmesan, sliced green onion for topping

Directions:

1. In a pot, heat oil over medium heat, while adding the onion and garlic. Then cook them for 4-5 minutes.
2. Add in the cauli and vegetable broth. Boil it and then cover for 15-20 minutes while covered.
3. Pour all contents of pot into a blender and season it.
4. Blend until smooth. Top it with your cheese and green onion.

Nutrition:
Calories: 37 kcal
Fats: 1 g
Carbs: 3 g
Protein: 3 g

THAI COCONUT SOUP

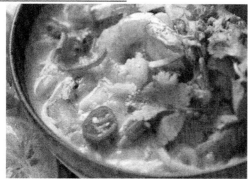

Preparation Time: 10 minutes
Cooking Time: 35 minutes
Servings: 4
Ingredients:

- 3 chicken breasts
- 9 oz. coconut milk
- 9 oz. chicken broth
- 2/3 tbsps. chili sauce

- 18 oz. water
- 2/3 tbsps. coconut aminos
- 2/3 oz. lime juice
- 2/3 tsps. ground ginger
- ¼ cup red boat fish sauce
- salt and pepper

Directions:

1. Slice up the chicken breasts thinly. Make them bite-sized.
2. In a large stock pot, mix your coconut milk, water, fish sauce, chili sauce, lime juice, ginger, coconut aminos, and broth. Bring to a boil.
3. Stir in chicken pieces. Then reduce the heat and cover pot, while simmering it for 30 minutes.
4. Remove the basil leaves and season it.

Nutrition:
Calories: 227 kcal Fats: 17 g
Carbs: 3 g Protein: 19 g

CHICKEN RAMEN SOUP

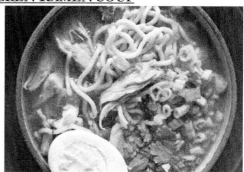

Preparation Time: 10 minutes
Cooking Time: 20 minutes
Servings: 2
Ingredients:

- 1 chicken breast
- 2 eggs
- 1 zucchini, made into noodles
- 4 cups chicken broth
- 2 cloves of garlic, peeled and minced
- 2 tbsps. coconut aminos
- 3 tbsps. avocado oil
- 1 tbsp. ginger

Directions:

1. Pan-fry the chicken in avocado oil in a pan until brown.
2. Hard boil your eggs and slice them in half.
3. Add chicken broth to a large pot and simmer with the garlic, coconut aminos, and ginger. Then add in the zucchini noodles for 4-5 minutes.
4. Put the broth into a bowl, top it with eggs and chicken slices, and season to your liking.

Nutrition:
Calories: 478 kcal Fats: 39 g
Carbs: 3 g Protein: 31 g

CHICKEN BROTH AND EGG DROP SOUP

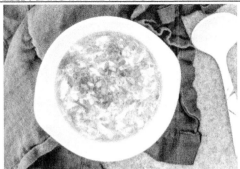

Preparation Time: 5 minutes
Cooking Time: 15 minutes
Servings: 2
Ingredients:

- 3 cups chicken broth
- 2 cups Swiss chard chopped
- 2 eggs, whisked
- 1 tsp. grated ginger
- 1 tsp. ground oregano
- 2 tbsps. coconut aminos
- salt and pepper

Directions:

1. Heat your broth in a saucepan.
2. Slowly drizzle in the eggs while stirring slowly.
3. Add the Swiss chard, grated ginger, oregano, and the coconut aminos. Next, season it and let it cook for 5-10 minutes.

Nutrition:
Calories: 225 kcal
Fats: 19 g
Carbs: 4 g
Protein: 11 g

OKRA AND BEEF STEW

Preparation Time: 15 minutes
Cooking Time: 25 minutes
Servings: 3 servings
Ingredients:

- 6 oz. okra, chopped
- 8 oz. beef sirloin, chopped
- 1 cup of water
- ¼ cup coconut cream
- 1 teaspoon dried basil
- ¼ teaspoon cumin seeds
- 1 tablespoon avocado oil

Directions:

1. Sprinkle the beef sirloin with cumin seeds and dried basil and put in the instant pot.
2. Add avocado oil and roast the meat on saute mode for 5 minutes. Stir it occasionally.
3. Then add coconut cream, water, and okra.
4. Close the lid and cook the stew on manual mode (high pressure) for 25 minutes. Allow the natural pressure release for 10 minutes.

Nutrition:
Calories 216
Fat 10.2 Fiber 2.5
Carbs 5.7 Protein 24.6

CHIPOTLE STEW

Preparation Time: 15 minutes
Cooking Time: 10 minutes
Servings: 3 servings
Ingredients:

- 2 chipotle chili in adobo sauce, chopped
- 1 oz. fresh cilantro, chopped
- 9 oz. chicken fillet, chopped
- 1 teaspoon ground paprika
- 2 tablespoons sesame seeds
- ¼ teaspoon salt
- 1 cup chicken broth

Directions:

1. In the mixing bowl mix up chipotle chili, cilantro, chicken fillet, ground paprika, sesame seeds, and salt.
2. Then transfer the Ingredients in the instant pot and add chicken broth.
3. Cook the stew on manual mode (high pressure) for 10 minutes. Allow the natural pressure release for 10 minutes more.

Nutrition:
Calories 230
Fat 10.6
Fiber 2.6
Carbs 4.5
Protein 27.6

KETO CHILI

Preparation Time: 10 minutes
Cooking Time: 25 minutes
Servings: 2 servings
Ingredients:

- ½ cup ground beef
- ½ teaspoon chili powder
- 1 teaspoon dried oregano
- ¼ cup crushed tomatoes
- 2 oz. scallions, diced
- 1 teaspoon avocado oil
- ¼ cup of water

Directions:

1. Mix up ground beef, chili powder, dried oregano, and scallions.
2. Then add avocado oil and stir the mixture.
3. Transfer it in the instant pot and cook on saute mode for 10 minutes.
4. Add water and crushed tomatoes. Stir the Ingredients with the help of the spatula until homogenous.
5. Close and seal the lid and cook the chili for 15 minutes on manual mode (high pressure). Then make a quick pressure release.

Nutrition:
Calories 94
Fat 4.6
Fiber 2.4
Carbs 5.6
Protein 8

PIZZA SOUP

Preparation Time: 10 minutes
Cooking Time: 22 minutes
Servings: 3 servings
Ingredients:

- ¼ cup cremini mushrooms, sliced
- 1 teaspoon tomato paste
- 4 oz. Mozzarella, shredded
- ½ jalapeno pepper, sliced
- ½ teaspoon Italian seasoning
- 1 teaspoon coconut oil
- 5 oz. Italian sausages, chopped
- 1 cup of water

Directions:

1. Melt the coconut oil in the instant pot on saute mode.
2. Add mushrooms and cook them for 10 minutes.
3. After this, add chopped sausages, Italian seasoning, sliced jalapeno, and tomato paste.
4. Mix up the Ingredients well and add water.
5. Close and seal the lid and cook the soup on manual mode (high pressure) for 12 minutes.
6. Then make a quick pressure release and ladle the soup in the bowls. Top it with Mozzarella.

Nutrition:
Calories 289
Fat 23.2
Fiber 0.2
Carbs 2.5
Protein 17.7

LAMB SOUP

Preparation Time: 10 minutes
Cooking Time: 25 minutes
Servings: 4 servings
Ingredients:

- ½ cup broccoli, roughly chopped
- 7 oz. lamb fillet, chopped
- ¼ teaspoon ground cumin
- ¼ daikon, chopped
- 2 bell peppers, chopped
- 1 tablespoon avocado oil
- 5 cups beef broth

Directions:

1. Saute the lamb fillet with avocado oil in the instant pot for 5 minutes.
2. Then add broccoli, ground cumin, and daikon, bell peppers, and beef broth.
3. Close and seal the lid.
4. Cook the soup on manual mode (high pressure) for 20 minutes.
5. Allow the natural pressure release.

Nutrition:
Calories 169 Fat 6
Fiber 1.3 Carbs 6.8 Protein 21

MINESTRONE SOUP

Preparation Time: 10 minutes
Cooking Time: 25 minutes
Servings: 4 servings
Ingredients:

- 1 ½ cup ground pork

- ½ bell pepper, chopped
- 2 tablespoons chives, chopped
- 2 oz. celery stalk, chopped
- 1 teaspoon butter
- 1 teaspoon Italian seasonings
- 4 cups chicken broth
- ½ cup mushrooms, sliced

Directions:

1. Heat up butter on the saute mode for 2 minutes.
2. Add bell pepper. Cook the vegetable for 5 minutes.
3. Then stir them well and add mushrooms, celery stalk, and Italian seasonings. Stir well and cook for 5 minutes more.
4. Add ground pork, chives, and chicken broth.
5. Close and seal the lid.
6. Cook the soup on manual mode (high pressure) for 15 minutes. Make a quick pressure release.

Nutrition:
Calories 408
Fat 27.2
Fiber 0.6
Carbs 3
Protein 35.6

CHORIZO SOUP

Preparation Time: 10 minutes
Cooking Time: 17 minutes
Servings: 3 servings
Ingredients:

- 8 oz. chorizo, chopped
- 1 teaspoon tomato paste
- 4 oz. scallions, diced
- 1 tablespoon dried cilantro
- ½ teaspoon chili powder
- 1 teaspoon avocado oil
- 2 cups beef broth

Directions:

1. Heat up avocado oil on saute mode for 1 minute.
2. Add chorizo and cook it for 6 minutes, stir it from time to time.
3. Then add scallions, tomato paste, cilantro, and chili powder. Stir well.
4. Add beef broth.
5. Close and seal the lid.
6. Cook the soup on manual mode (high pressure) for 10 minutes. Make a quick pressure release.

Nutrition:
Calories 387
Fat 30.2
Fiber 1.3
Carbs 5.5
Protein 22.3

RED FETA SOUP

Preparation Time: 10 minutes
Cooking Time: 25 minutes
Servings: 4 servings
Ingredients:

- 1 cup broccoli, chopped
- 1 teaspoon tomato paste
- ½ cup coconut cream

- 4 cups beef broth
- 1 teaspoon chili flakes
- 6 oz. feta, crumbled

Directions:

1. Put broccoli, tomato paste, coconut cream, and beef broth in the instant pot.
2. Add chili flakes and stir the mixture until it is red.
3. Then close and seal the lid and cook the soup for 8 minutes on manual mode (high pressure).
4. Then make a quick pressure release and open the lid.
5. Add feta cheese and saute the soup on saute mode for 5 minutes more.

Nutrition:
Calories 229
Fat 17.7
Fiber 1.3
Carbs 6.1
Protein 12.3

"RAMEN" SOUP

Preparation Time: 10 minutes
Cooking Time: 15 minutes
Servings: 2 servings
Ingredients:

- 1 zucchini, trimmed
- 2 cups chicken broth
- 2 eggs, boiled, peeled
- 1 tablespoon coconut aminos
- 5 oz. beef loin, strips
- 1 teaspoon chili flakes
- 1 tablespoon chives, chopped
- ½ teaspoon salt

Directions:

1. Put the beef loin strips in the instant pot.
2. Add chili flakes, salt, and chicken broth.
3. Close and seal the lid. Cook the **Ingredients:** on manual mode (high pressure) for 15 minutes. Make a quick pressure release and open the lid.
4. Then make the s from zucchini with the help of the spiralizer and add them in the soup.
5. Add chives and coconut aminos.
6. Then ladle the soup in the bowls and top with halved eggs.

Nutrition:
Calories 254
Fat 11.8
Fiber 1.1
Carbs 6.2
Protein 30.6

BEEF TAGINE

Preparation Time: 15 minutes
Cooking Time: 25 minutes
Servings: 6 servings
Ingredients:

- 1-pound beef fillet, chopped
- 1 eggplant, chopped
- 6 oz. scallions, chopped
- 1 teaspoon ground allspices
- 1 teaspoon Erythritol

- 1 teaspoon coconut oil
- 4 cups beef broth

Directions:

1. Put all Ingredients in the instant pot.
2. Close and seal the lid.
3. Cook the meal on manual mode (high pressure) for 25 minutes.
4. Then allow the natural pressure release for 15 minutes.

Nutrition:
Calories 146
Fat 5.3
Fiber 3.5
Carbs 8.8
Protein 16.7

TOMATILLOS FISH STEW

Preparation Time: 15 minutes
Cooking Time: 12 minutes
Servings: 2 servings
Ingredients:

- 2 tomatillos, chopped
- 10 oz. salmon fillet, chopped
- 1 teaspoon ground paprika
- ½ teaspoon ground turmeric
- 1 cup coconut cream
- ½ teaspoon salt

Directions:

1. Put all Ingredients in the instant pot.
2. Close and seal the lid.
3. Cook the fish stew on manual mode (high pressure) for 12 minutes.
4. Then allow the natural pressure release for 10 minutes.

Nutrition:
Calories 479
Fat 37.9
Fiber 3.8
Carbs 9.6
Protein 30.8

CHILI VERDE SOUP

Preparation Time: 10 minutes
Cooking Time: 25 minutes
Servings: 4 servings
Ingredients:

- 2 oz. chili Verde sauce
- ½ cup Cheddar cheese, shredded
- 5 cups chicken broth
- 1-pound chicken breast, skinless, boneless
- 1 tablespoon dried cilantro

Directions:

1. Put chicken breast and chicken broth in the instant pot.
2. Add cilantro, close and seal the lid.
3. Then cook the Ingredients on manual (high pressure) for 15 minutes.
4. Make a quick pressure release and open the li.
5. Shred the chicken breast with the help of the fork.
6. Add dried cilantro and chili Verde sauce in the soup and cook it on saute mode for 10 minutes.

7. Then add dried cilantro and stir well.

Nutrition:
Calories 257
Fat 10.2
Fiber 0.2
Carbs 4
Protein 34.5

PEPPER STUFFING SOUP

Preparation Time: 10 minutes
Cooking Time: 14 minutes
Servings: 4 servings
Ingredients:

- 1 cup ground beef
- ½ cup cauliflower, shredded
- 1 teaspoon dried oregano
- ½ teaspoon salt
- 1 teaspoon tomato paste
- 1 teaspoon minced garlic
- 4 cups of water
- ¼ cup of coconut milk

Directions:

1. Put all Ingredients in the instant pot bowl and stir well.
2. Then close and seal the lid.
3. Cook the soup on manual mode (high pressure) for 14 minutes.
4. When the time of cooking is finished, make a quick pressure release and open the lid.

Nutrition:
Calories 106
Fat 7.7
Fiber 0.9
Carbs 2.2
Protein 7.3

STEAK SOUP

Preparation Time: 10 minutes
Cooking Time: 40 minutes
Servings: 5 servings
Ingredients:

- 5 oz. scallions, diced
- 1 tablespoon coconut oil
- 1 oz. daikon, diced
- 1-pound beef round steak, chopped
- 1 teaspoon dried thyme
- 5 cups of water
- ½ teaspoon ground black pepper

Directions:

1. Heat up coconut oil on saute mode for 2 minutes.
2. Add daikon and scallions.
3. After this, stir them well and add chopped beef steak, thyme, and ground black pepper.
4. Saute the Ingredients for 5 minutes more and then add water.
5. Close and seal the lid.
6. Cook the soup on manual mode (high pressure) for 35 minutes. Make a quick pressure release.

Nutrition:
Calories 232 Fat 11
Fiber 0.9 Carbs 2.5 Protein 29.5

MEAT SPINACH STEW

Preparation Time: 20 minutes
Cooking Time: 30 minutes
Servings: 4 servings
Ingredients:

- 2 cups spinach, chopped
- 1-pound beef sirloin, chopped
- 1 teaspoon allspices
- 3 cups chicken broth
- 1 cup of coconut milk
- 1 teaspoon coconut aminos

Directions:

1. Put all Ingredients in the instant pot.
2. Close and seal the lid.
3. After this, set the manual mode (high pressure) and cook the stew for 30 minutes.
4. When the cooking time is finished, allow the natural pressure release for 10 minutes.
5. Stir the stew gently before serving.

Nutrition:
Calories 383
Fat 22.2
Fiber 1.8
Carbs 5.1
Protein 39.9

LEEK SOUP

Preparation Time: 10 minutes
Cooking Time: 15 minutes
Servings: 4 servings
Ingredients:

- 7 oz. leek, chopped
- 2 oz. Monterey Jack cheese, shredded
- 1 teaspoon Italian seasonings
- ½ teaspoon salt
- 4 tablespoons butter
- 2 cups chicken broth

Directions:

1. Heat up butter in the instant pot for 4 minutes.
2. Then add chopped leek, salt, and Italian seasonings.
3. Cook the leek on saute mode for 5 minutes. Stir the vegetables from time to time.
4. After this, add chicken broth and close the lid.
5. Cook the soup on saute mode for 10 minutes.
6. Then add shredded cheese and stir it till the cheese is melted.
7. The soup is cooked.

Nutrition:
Calories 208
Fat 17
Fiber 0.9
Carbs 7.7
Protein 6.8

ASPARAGUS SOUP

Preparation Time: 10 minutes
Cooking Time: 17 minutes
Servings: 4 servings
Ingredients:

- 1 cup asparagus, chopped
- 2 cups of coconut milk

- 1 teaspoon salt
- ½ teaspoon cayenne pepper
- 3 oz. scallions, diced
- 1 teaspoon olive oil

Directions:
1. Saute the chopped asparagus, scallions, and olive oil in the instant pot for 7 minutes.
2. Then stir the vegetables well and add cayenne pepper, salt, and coconut milk
3. Cook the soup on manual mode (high pressure) for 10 minutes.
4. After this, make a quick pressure release and open the lid.
5. Blend the soup until you get the creamy texture.

Nutrition:
Calories 300 Fat 29.9
Fiber 4 Carbs 9.6 Protein 3.9

Bok Choy Soup

Preparation Time: 5 minutes
Cooking Time: 2 minutes
Servings: 1 serving
Ingredients:
- 1 bok choy stalk, chopped
- ¼ teaspoon nutritional yeast
- ½ teaspoon onion powder
- ¼ teaspoon chili flakes
- 1 cup chicken broth

Directions:
1. Put all Ingredients from the list above in the instant pot.
2. Close and seal the lid and cook the soup on manual (high pressure) for 2 minutes.
3. Make a quick pressure release.

Nutrition:
Calories 58
Fat 1.7
Fiber 1.3
Carbs 4.5
Protein 6.9

Curry Kale Soup

Preparation Time: 10 minutes
Cooking Time: 15 minutes
Servings: 3 servings
Ingredients:
- 2 cups kale
- 1 tablespoon fresh cilantro
- 1 teaspoon curry paste
- ½ cup heavy cream
- ½ cup ground chicken
- 1 teaspoon almond butter
- ½ teaspoon salt 1 cup chicken stock

Directions:
1. Blend the kale until smooth and put it in the instant pot.
2. Add cilantro, almond butter, and ground chicken. Saute the mixture for 5 minutes.
3. Meanwhile, in the shallow bowl, mix up curry paste and heavy cream. When the liquid is smooth, pour it in the instant pot.

4. Add chicken stock and salt, and close the lid.
5. Cook the soup on manual (high pressure) for 10 minutes. Make a quick pressure release.

Nutrition:
Calories 183
Fat 13.3
Fiber 1.2
Carbs 7
Protein 9.9

Turmeric Rutabaga Soup

Preparation Time: 15 minutes
Cooking Time: 15 minutes
Servings: 5 servings
Ingredients:
- 3 turnips, chopped
- 1 teaspoon ginger paste
- 2 oz. celery, chopped
- 1 teaspoon ground turmeric
- 1 teaspoon minced garlic
- 2 cups of coconut milk
- 1 cup beef broth
- 2 oz. bell pepper, chopped

Directions:
1. Place all Ingredients in the instant pot and stir them gently.
2. Then close and seal the lid; set manual mode (high pressure) and cook the soup for 15 minutes.
3. Then allow the natural pressure release for 10 minutes and ladle the soup into the serving bowls.

Nutrition:
Calories 255
Fat 23.2
Fiber 3.6
Carbs 11.4
Protein 4

Cream of Mushrooms Soup

Preparation Time: 10 minutes
Cooking Time: 35 minutes
Servings: 6 servings
Ingredients:
- 3 cups cremini mushrooms, sliced
- 1 cup of coconut milk
- 1 tablespoon almond flour
- 1 teaspoon salt
- 1 teaspoon ground black pepper
- 4 cups chicken broth
- 3 tablespoons butter

Directions:
1. Melt the butter on saute mode.
2. Add cremini mushrooms and saute them for 10 minutes. Stir them with the help of the spatula from time to time.
3. After this, in the bowl mix up salt, almond flour, and ground black pepper. Add coconut milk and stir the liquid.
4. Pour the liquid over the mushrooms.
5. Add chicken broth. Close and seal the lid.

6. Cook the soup on saute mode for 25 minutes.

Nutrition:
Calories 206
Fat 18.6
Fiber 1.7
Carbs 5.5
Protein 6.2

FLU SOUP

Preparation Time: 10 minutes
Cooking Time: 15 minutes
Servings: 4 servings
Ingredients:

- 1 cup mushrooms, chopped
- 1 cup spinach, chopped
- 3 oz. scallions, diced
- 2 oz. Cheddar cheese, shredded
- 1 teaspoon cayenne pepper
- 1 cup organic almond milk
- 2 cups chicken broth
- ½ teaspoon salt

Directions:

1. Put all Ingredients in the instant pot and close the lid.
2. Set the manual mode (high pressure) and cook the soup for 15 minutes.
3. Make a quick pressure release.
4. Blend the soup with the help of the immersion blender.
5. When the soup will get smooth texture – it is cooked.

Nutrition:
Calories 228 Fat 19.9 Fiber 2.3
Carbs 6.6 Protein 8.5

JALAPENO SOUP

Preparation Time: 10 minutes
Cooking Time: 10 minutes
Servings: 4 servings
Ingredients:

- 2 jalapeno peppers, sliced
- 3 oz. pancetta, chopped
- ½ cup heavy cream
- 2 cups of water
- ½ cup Monterey jack cheese, shredded
- ½ teaspoon garlic powder
- 1 teaspoon coconut oil
- ½ teaspoon smoked paprika

Directions:

1. Toss pancetta in the instant pot, add coconut oil and cook it for 4 minutes on saute mode. Stir it from time to time.
2. After this, add sliced jalapenos, garlic powder, and smoked paprika.
3. Stir the Ingredients for 1 minute.
4. Add heavy cream and water.
5. Then add Monterey Jack cheese and stir the soup well.
6. Close and seal the lid; cook the soup for 5 minutes on manual mode (high pressure); make a quick pressure release.

Nutrition:
Calories 234
Fat 20
Fiber 0.4
Carbs 1.7
Protein 11.8

GARDEN SOUP

Preparation Time: 20 minutes
Cooking Time: 29 minutes
Servings: 5 servings
Ingredients:

- ½ cup cauliflower florets
- 1 cup kale, chopped
- 1 garlic clove, diced
- 1 tablespoon olive oil
- 1 teaspoon sea salt
- 6 cups beef broth
- 2 tablespoons chives, chopped

Directions:

1. Heat up olive oil in the instant pot on saute mode for 2 minutes and add clove.
2. Cook the vegetables for 2 minutes and stir well.
3. Add kale, cauliflower, and sea salt, chives, and beef broth.
4. Close and seal the lid.
5. Cook the soup on manual mode (high pressure) for 5 minutes.
6. Then make a quick pressure release and open the lid.
7. Ladle the soup into the bowls.

Nutrition:
Calories 80 Fat 4.5
Fiber 0.5 Carbs 2.3 Protein 6.5

SHIRATAKI NOODLE SOUP

Preparation Time: 25 minutes
Cooking Time: 15 minutes
Servings: 2 servings
Ingredients:

- 2 oz. shirataki noodles
- 2 cups of water
- 6 oz. chicken fillet, chopped
- 1 teaspoon salt
- 1 tablespoon coconut aminos

Directions:

1. Pour water in the instant pot bowl.
2. Add salt and chopped chicken fillet. Close and seal the lid.
3. Cook the Ingredients on manual mode (high pressure) for 15 minutes. Allow the natural pressure release for 10 minutes.
4. After this, add shirataki noodles and coconut aminos.
5. Leave the soup for 10 minutes to rest.

Nutrition:
Calories 175 Fat 6.3
Fiber 3 Carbs 1.5
Protein 24.8

CORDON BLUE SOUP

Preparation Time: 15 minutes
Cooking Time: 6 minutes
Servings: 4 servings
Ingredients:
- 4 cups chicken broth
- 7 oz. ham, chopped
- 3 oz. Mozzarella cheese, shredded
- 1 teaspoon ground black pepper
- ½ teaspoon salt
- 2 tablespoons ricotta cheese
- 2 oz. scallions, chopped

Directions:
1. Put all Ingredients in the instant pot bowl and stir gently.
2. Close and seal the lid; cook the soup on manual mode (high pressure) for 6 minutes.
3. Then allow the natural pressure release for 10 minutes and ladle the soup into the bowls.

Nutrition:
Calories 196
Fat 10.1
Fiber 1.2
Carbs 5.3
Protein 20.3

BACON SOUP

Preparation Time: 10 minutes
Cooking Time: 20 minutes
Servings: 4 servings
Ingredients:
- 3 oz. bacon, chopped
- 1 cup cheddar cheese, shredded
- 1 tablespoon scallions, chopped
- 3 cups beef broth 1 cup of coconut milk
- 1 teaspoon curry powder

Directions:
1. Heat up the instant pot on saute mode for 3 minutes and add bacon.
2. Cook it for 5 minutes. Stir it from time to time.
3. Then add scallions and curry powder. Cook the Ingredients for 5 minutes more. Stir them from time to time.
4. After this, add coconut milk and beef broth.
5. Add cheddar cheese and stir the soup well.
6. Cook it on manual mode (high pressure) for 10 minutes. Make a quick pressure release.
7. Mix up the soup well before serving.

Nutrition:
calories 398 fat 33.6 fiber 1.5
carbs 5.1 protein 20

PAPRIKA ZUCCHINI SOUP

Preparation Time: 10 minutes
Cooking Time: 1 minute
Servings: 2 servings
Ingredients:
- 1 zucchini, grated
- 1 teaspoon ground paprika
- ½ teaspoon cayenne pepper
- ½ cup of coconut milk
- 1 cup beef broth

- 1 tablespoon dried cilantro
- 1 oz. Parmesan, grated

Directions:
1. Put the grated zucchini, paprika, cayenne pepper, coconut milk, beef broth, and dried cilantro in the instant pot.
2. Close and seal the lid.
3. Cook the soup on manual (high pressure) for 1 minute. Make a quick pressure release.
4. Ladle the soup in the serving bowls and top with parmesan.

Nutrition:
calories 223
fat 18.4
fiber 2.9
carbs 8.4
protein 9.7

EGG DROP SOUP

Preparation Time: 5 minutes
Cooking Time: 10 minutes
Servings: 4 servings
Ingredients:
- 4 cups chicken broth
- 2 tablespoons fresh dill, chopped
- 2 eggs, beaten
- 1 teaspoon salt

Directions:
1. Pour chicken broth in the instant pot.
2. Add salt and bring it to boil on Saute mode.
3. Then add beaten eggs and stir the liquid well.
4. Add dill and saute it for 5 minutes.
5. The soup is cooked.

Nutrition:
calories 74
fat 3.6
fiber 0.2
carbs 2
protein 7.9

BUFFALO STYLE SOUP

Preparation Time: 7 minutes
Cooking Time: 10 minutes
Servings: 2 servings
Ingredients:
- 6 oz. chicken, cooked
- 2 oz. Mozzarella, shredded
- 4 tablespoons coconut milk
- ¼ teaspoon white pepper
- ¾ teaspoon salt
- 2 tablespoons keto Buffalo sauce
- 1 oz. celery stalk, chopped
- 1 cup of water

Directions:
1. Place the chopped celery stalk, water, salt, white pepper, coconut milk, and Mozzarella in the instant pot. Stir it gently.
2. Set the "Manual" mode (High pressure) and turn on the timer for 7 minutes.
3. Shred the cooked chicken and combine it together with Buffalo Sauce.

4. Make quick pressure release and transfer the soup on the bowls.
5. Add shredded chicken and stir it.

Nutrition:
calories 287
fat 14.8
fiber 1.5
carbs 4.3
protein 33.5

CHAPTER 15:

POULTRY

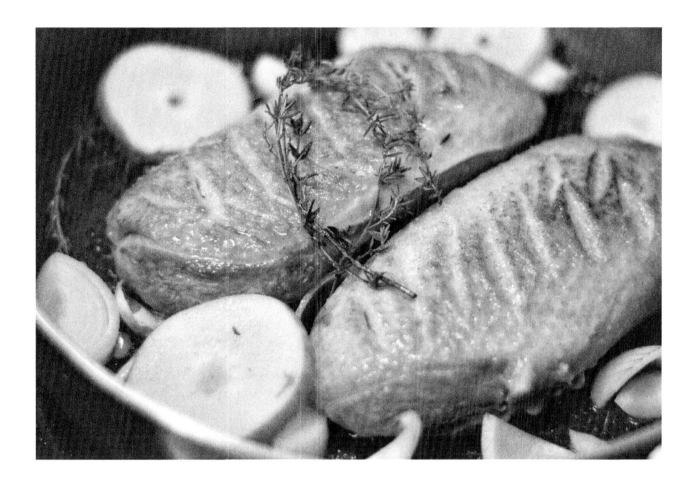

ONE-POT ITALIAN CHICKEN
INGREDIENTS
- One tablespoon olive oil
- 20g butter
- Four small chicken breasts fillets
- Two garlic cloves, finely chopped
- 80g (1/2 cup) sun-dried tomatoes, sliced
- 80ml (1/3 cup) white wine
- 250ml (1 cup) thickened cream
- 125ml (1/2 cup) Massel chicken style liquid stock
- 60g pkt baby spinach
- 1 cup fresh basil leaves, torn
- Crusty bread, to serve

METHOD
In a large non-stick frying dish, heat the oil and butter over high heat until butter is foamy. Season and add the chicken to the pot. Reduce to medium-high heat.
Cook the chicken on each side for 5 minutes until cooked. Move to board. Switch to board. To keep warm, cover with foil.
In the pan, put the garlic.
Cook, stirring, or until aromatic for 1 minute. Stir in the tomatoes and cover. Add wine and cook until reduced for 1 minute.
Stir in the cream and stock. Return the chicken to the bowl and cook for 5 minutes or until liquid has decreased.
Cut the spinach until it wilts. Spray the basil leaves season and spray. Serve with bread crusty.

KETO CHICKEN PARMI BOWL
INGREDIENTS
- One egg
- 80g (2/3 cup) almond meal
- 40g (1/2 cup) finely grated parmesan
- Two tablespoons finely chopped fresh continental parsley, plus extra to serve
- 4 x (about 125g each) chicken breast schnitzels (uncrumbed)
- Extra virgin olive oil, to shallow fry, plus extra to drizzle
- 80ml (1/3 cup) tomato pasta sauce
- Four slices smoked ham
- 50g (1/2 cup) coarsely grated fresh mozzarella
- 1.1kg (1 head) cauliflower, trimmed, cut into florets
- 25g butter
- 125ml (1/2 cup) thickened cream
- White pepper, to season
- One tablespoon chopped fresh chives, optional

METHOD
In a shallow cup, whisk the egg gently. On a plate blend the meal of the almond, parmesan and parsley. Feed poultry. Feed poultry. Dip one chicken piece into an egg and press to coat into the almond meal mixture. Switch to a tray lined.

Repeat with the remaining meal mixture of rice, egg and almond. Put 30 minutes to rest in the fridge.
In the purée, put the cauliflower over high heat and cover with water in a medium casserole. Cook 15-20 minutes or tenderly. Drain into a pot, and book 1/3 of a cup of liquid. Steam the butter in the pan over medium heat until it is sprayed. Add the cooked coolant, milk and liquid reserved for cooking. Simmer for 3 minutes or until slightly reduced. Remove from heat and mix with a stab mixer until smooth. Top with white pepper and salt.
Cut the cabbage, if used. Cover and hold.
Heat 1 cm of oil over high heat in a big, heavy-duty fry. Cook the chicken in batches, on each side for three minutes, or until golden and crisp. Clear from the tray the bakery paper. Move to the tray the chicken.
Preheat up the barbecue. Spoon each schnitzel with a dollop of tomato pasta sauce. Sprinkle with ham and cheese. Grill for 3-4 minutes or for golden cheese. When necessary, sprinkle with extra parsley.
In the meantime, return to medium heat and cook the cauliflower puree, stir for 2 minutes or until cooked. Serve the puree with the chicken.

CREAMY CHICKEN, BACON AND CAULIFLOWER BAKE
INGREDIENTS
- 1 tablespoon olive oil
- 10g butter
- One small (900g) cauliflower, trimmed, cut into small florets
- Two rashers (120g) bacon, chopped
- One bunch English spinach, trimmed, chopped
- 125ml (1/2 cup) pouring cream
- Two teaspoons fresh thyme leaves (optional)
- Two green shallots, trimmed, sliced
- 500g Lilydale Free Range Chicken Thigh, fat trimmed
- 55g (1/2 cup) 3-cheese mix

METHOD
Preheat oven forced to 200C/180C fan. Grate a 2L (8-cup) ovenproof bakery lightly.
In a large frying pot heat, oil and butter over medium until the butter is moistened. Add the bacon and the cauliflower. Cook for 8-10 minutes, stirring regularly, or until lightly golden.
Remove the spinach to the saucepan. Cook for two minutes, stirring, or until wilted. Remove the milk, thyme and half of the shallot from the oil. Delete to merge. Transfer to the dish prepared.
Clean the pan and brush with oil. Attach the chicken to the pan and cook on both sides for about 2 minutes or until golden. Place on top of the mixture of the cauliflower.
Sprinkle the chicken with cheese. Bake until golden for 20-25 minutes. Stand 5 minutes until the remaining shallot is served.

BAKED CHICKEN WITH TARRAGON AND CREAM

INGREDIENTS

- One tablespoon extra-virgin olive oil
- 4 (about 1.2kg) chicken Marylands
- 15g butter
- One large red onion halved, cut into thin wedges
- 80ml (1/3 cup) dry white wine
- 80ml (1/3 cup) Massel salt reduced chicken style liquid stock
- 300g (2 cups) frozen broad beans
- 80ml (1/3 cup) pouring cream
- 1/3 cup fresh tarragon leaves, plus extra, to serve

METHOD

Preheat oven forced to 200C/180C fan. Heat half the oil over medium heat in a big, flameproof, ovenproof pan. Feed poultry. Feed poultry. Cook for 4-5 minutes or until golden, skin-side down. Turn and cook 2 minutes longer. Move to board. Switch to board. Pour the fat out of the bowl and dump it. Heat the remaining butter and oil over medium-low heat in the pan. Cook onion, turn, 2 minutes or golden. Add the wine. Add the wine. Boil 1 minute. Simmer. Add stock. Add stock. Boil 1 minute. Boil. Remove from fire. Remove from heat. Place the chicken on the onion. Bake for 30 minutes or until chicken has been cooked. Switch the oven off. Fill a bakery tray with pastry paper. Move the chicken to the plate. Place warm in the oven.

In the meantime, put the big beans in a heat resistant dish. Boiling water shell. Sheet. Stand 2 minutes. Wait 2 minutes. Drain. Drain. Cool under cold running water. Cool. Peel. Peel. Back to medium humidity. Bring to a frying pan. Simmer until slightly reduced or for 2 minutes. Add milk. Add butter. Simmer 2-3 minutes, or thicken slightly. Attach the tarragon. Attach the tarragon. Boil 1 minute. Boil. Remove from fire. Remove from heat. Stir the big beans in two-thirds. Go back to the pan chicken. Sprinkle with other broad beans and extra tarragon.

COUNTRY-STYLE CHICKEN STEW

Preparation Time: 20 minutes
Cooking Time: 1 hour
Servings: 6
Ingredients:

- 1 pound chicken thighs
- 2 tablespoons butter, room temperature
- 1/2 pound carrots, chopped
- 1 bell pepper, chopped
- 1 chile pepper, deveined and minced
- 1 cup tomato puree
- Kosher salt and ground black pepper, to taste
- 1/2 teaspoon smoked paprika
- 1 onion, finely chopped
- 1 teaspoon garlic, sliced
- 4 cups vegetable broth
- 1 teaspoon dried basil
- 1 celery, chopped

Directions:

1. Melt the butter in a stockpot over medium-high flame. Sweat the onion and garlic until just tender and fragrant.
2. Reduce the heat to medium-low. Stir in the broth, chicken thighs, and basil; bring to a rolling boil.
3. Add in the remaining Ingredients. Partially cover and let it simmer for 45 to 50 minutes. Shred the meat, discarding the bones; add the chicken back to the pot.

Nutrition:
280 Calories 14.7g Fat
2.5g Carbs 25.6g Protein
2.5g Fiber

AUTUMN CHICKEN SOUP WITH ROOT VEGETABLES

Preparation Time: 10 minutes
Cooking Time: 25 minutes
Servings: 4
Ingredients: 4 cups chicken broth

- 1 cup full-fat milk
- 1 cup double cream
- 1/2 cup turnip, chopped
- 2 chicken drumsticks, boneless and cut into small pieces
- Salt and pepper, to taste
- 1 tablespoon butter
- 1 teaspoon garlic, finely minced
- 1 carrot, chopped
- 1/2 parsnip, chopped
- 1/2 celery - 1 whole egg

Directions:

1. Melt the butter in a heavy-bottomed pot over medium-high heat; sauté the garlic until aromatic or about 1 minute. Add in the vegetables and continue to cook until they've softened.
2. Add in the chicken and cook until it is no longer pink for about 4 minutes. Season with salt and pepper.
3. Pour in the chicken broth, milk, and heavy cream and bring it to a boil.
4. Reduce the heat to. Partially cover and continue to simmer for 20 to 25 minutes longer. Afterwards, fold the beaten egg and stir until it is well incorporated.

Nutrition: 342 Calories 22.4g Fat
6.3g Carbs 25.2g Protein 1.3g Fiber

PANNA COTTA WITH CHICKEN AND BLEU D' AUVERGNE

Preparation Time: 10 minutes
Cooking Time: 20 minutes
Servings:
Ingredients:

- 2 chicken legs, boneless and skinless
- 1 tablespoon avocado oil
- 2 teaspoons granular erythritol
- 3 tablespoons water
- 1 cup Bleu d' Auvergne, crumbled
- 2 gelatin sheets
- 3/4 cup double cream

- Salt and cayenne pepper, to your liking

Directions:

1. Heat the oil in a frying pan over medium-high heat; fry the chicken for about 10 minutes.
2. Soak the gelatin sheets in cold water. Cook with the cream, erythritol, water, and Bleu d' Auvergne.
3. Season with salt and pepper and let it simmer over the low heat, stirring for about 3 minutes. Spoon the mixture into four ramekins.

Nutrition:

306 Calories
18.3g Fat
4.7g Carbs
29.5g Protein
0g Fiber

BREADED CHICKEN FILLETS

Preparation Time: 15 minutes
Cooking Time: 30 minutes
Servings: 4
Ingredients:

- 1 pound chicken fillets
- 3 bell peppers, quartered lengthwise
- 1/3 cup Romano cheese
- 2 teaspoons olive oil
- 1 garlic clove, minced
- Kosher salt and ground black pepper, to taste
- 1/3 cup crushed pork rinds

Directions:

1. Start by preheating your oven to 410 degrees F.
2. Mix the crushed pork rinds, Romano cheese, olive oil and minced garlic. Dredge the chicken into this mixture.
3. Place the chicken in a lightly greased baking dish. Season with salt and black pepper to taste.
4. Scatter the peppers around the chicken and bake in the preheated oven for 20 to 25 minutes or until thoroughly cooked.

Nutrition:

367 Calories
16.9g Fat
6g Carbs
43g Protein
0.7g Fiber

CHICKEN DRUMSTICKS WITH BROCCOLI AND CHEESE

Preparation Time: 40 minutes
Cooking Time: 1 hour 15 minutes
Servings: 4
Ingredients:

- 1 pound chicken drumsticks
- 1 pound broccoli, broken into florets
- 2 cups cheddar cheese, shredded
- 1/2 teaspoon dried oregano
- 1/2 teaspoon dried basil
- 3 tablespoons olive oil
- 1 celery, sliced
- 1 cup green onions, chopped
- 1 teaspoon minced green garlic

Directions:

1. Roast the chicken drumsticks in the preheated oven at 380 degrees F for 30 to 35 minutes. Add in the broccoli, celery, green onions, and green garlic.
2. Add in the oregano, basil and olive oil; roast an additional 15 minutes.

Nutrition:

533 Calories
40.2g Fat
5.4g Carbs
35.1g Protein
3.5g Fiber

TURKEY HAM AND MOZZARELLA PATE

Preparation Time: 5 minutes
Cooking Time: 10 minutes
Servings: 6
Ingredients:

- 4 ounces turkey ham, chopped
- 2 tablespoons fresh parsley, roughly chopped
- 2 tablespoons flaxseed meal
- 4 ounces mozzarella cheese, crumbled
- 2 tablespoons sunflower seeds

Directions:

1. Thoroughly combine the Ingredients, except for the sunflower seeds, in your food processor.
2. Spoon the mixture into a serving bowl and scatter the sunflower seeds over the top.

Nutrition:

212 Calories
18.8g Fat
2g Carbs
10.6g Protein
1.6g Fiber

GREEK-STYLE SAUCY CHICKEN DRUMETTES

Preparation Time: 25 minutes
Cooking Time: 50 minutes
Servings: 6
Ingredients:

- 1 ½ pounds chicken drumettes
- 1/2 cup port wine
- 1/2 cup onions, chopped
- 2 garlic cloves, minced
- 1 teaspoon tzatziki spice mix
- 1 cup double cream
- 2 tablespoons butter
- Sea salt and crushed mixed peppercorns, to season

Directions:

1. Melt the butter in an oven-proof skillet over a moderate heat; then, cook the chicken for about 8 minutes.
2. Add in the onions, garlic, wine, tzatziki spice mix, double cream, salt, and pepper.
3. Bake in the preheated oven at 390 degrees F for 35 to 40 minutes (a meat thermometer should register 165 degrees F).

Nutrition:

333 Calories 20.2g Fat
2g Carbs 33.5g Protein 0.2g Fiber

CHICKEN WITH AVOCADO SAUCE

Preparation Time: 10 minutes
Cooking Time: 20 minutes
Servings: 4
Ingredients:

- 8 chicken wings, boneless, cut into bite-size chunks
- 2 tablespoons olive oil
- Sea salt and pepper, to your liking
- 2 eggs
- 1 teaspoon onion powder
- 1 teaspoon hot paprika
- 1/3 teaspoon mustard seeds
- 1/3 cup almond meal

For the Sauce:

- 1/2 cup mayonnaise
- 1/2 medium avocado
- 1/2 teaspoon sea salt
- 1 teaspoon green garlic, minced

Directions:

1. Pat dry the chicken wings with a paper towel.
2. Thoroughly combine the almond meal, salt, pepper, onion powder, paprika, and mustard seeds.
3. Whisk the eggs in a separate dish. Dredge the chicken chunks into the whisked eggs, then in the almond meal mixture.
4. In a frying pan, heat the oil over a moderate heat; once hot, fry the chicken for about 10 minutes, stirring continuously to ensure even cooking.
5. Make the sauce by whisking all of the sauce Ingredients.

Nutrition:
370 Calories
25g Fat
4.1g Carbs
31.4g Protein
2.6g Fiber

OLD-FASHIONED TURKEY CHOWDER

Preparation Time: 15 minutes
Cooking Time: 35 minutes
Servings: 4
Ingredients:

- 2 tablespoons olive oil
- 2 tablespoons yellow onions, chopped
- 2 cloves garlic, roughly chopped
- 1/2 pound leftover roast turkey, shredded and skin removed
- 1 teaspoon Mediterranean spice mix
- 3 cups chicken bone broth
- 1 ½ cups milk
- 1/2 cup double cream
- 1 egg, lightly beaten
- 2 tablespoons dry sherry

Directions:

1. Heat the olive oil in a heavy-bottomed pot over a moderate flame. Sauté the onion and garlic until they've softened.
2. Stir in the leftover roast turkey, Mediterranean spice mix, and chicken bone broth; bring to a rapid boil. Partially cover and continue to cook for 20 to 25 minutes.
3. Turn the heat to simmer. Pour in the milk and double cream and continue to cook until it has reduced slightly.
4. Fold in the egg and dry sherry; continue to simmer, stirring frequently, for a further 2 minutes.

Nutrition:
350 Calories
25.8g Fat
5.5g Carbs
20g Protein
0.1g Fiber

DUCK AND EGGPLANT CASSEROLE

Preparation Time: 10 minutes
Cooking Time: 45 minutes
Servings: 4
Ingredients:

- 1 pound ground duck meat
- 1 ½ tablespoons ghee, melted
- 1/3 cup double cream
- 1/2 pound eggplant, peeled and sliced
- 1 ½ cups almond flour
- Salt and black pepper, to taste
- 1/2 teaspoon fennel seeds
- 1/2 teaspoon oregano, dried
- 8 eggs

Directions:

1. Mix the almond flour with salt, black, fennel seeds, and oregano. Fold in one egg and the melted ghee and whisk to combine well.
2. Press the crust into the bottom of a lightly-oiled pie pan. Cook the ground duck until no longer pink for about 3 minutes, stirring continuously.
3. Whisk the remaining eggs and double cream. Fold in the browned meat and stir until everything is well incorporated. Pour the mixture into the prepared crust. Top with the eggplant slices.
4. Bake for about 40 minutes. Cut into four pieces.

Nutrition:
562 Calories
49.5g Fat
6.7g Carbs
22.5g Protein
2.1g Fiber

HERBED CHICKEN BREASTS

Preparation Time: 10 minutes
Cooking Time: 40 minutes
Servings: 8
Ingredients:

- 4 chicken breasts, skinless and boneless
- 1 Italian pepper, deveined and thinly sliced
- 10 black olives, pitted
- 1 ½ cups vegetable broth
- 2 garlic cloves, pressed
- 2 tablespoons olive oil
- 1 tablespoon Old Sub Sailor
- Salt, to taste

Directions:

1. Rub the chicken with the garlic and Old Sub Sailor; salt to taste. Heat the oil in a frying pan over a moderately high heat.
2. Sear the chicken until it is browned on all sides, about 5 minutes.
3. Add in the pepper, olives, and vegetable broth and bring it to boil. Reduce the heat simmer and continue to cook, partially covered, for 30 to 35 minutes.

Nutrition:
306 Calories
17.8g Fat
3.1g Carbs
31.7g Protein
0.2g Fiber

CHEESE AND PROSCIUTTO CHICKEN ROULADE

Preparation Time: 15 minutes
Cooking Time: 35 minutes
Servings: 2
Ingredients:

- 1/2 cup Ricotta cheese
- 4 slices of prosciutto
- 1 pound chicken fillet
- 1 tablespoon fresh coriander, chopped
- Salt and ground black pepper, to taste pepper
- 1 teaspoon cayenne pepper

Directions:

1. Season the chicken fillet with salt and pepper. Spread the Ricotta cheese over the chicken fillet; sprinkle with the fresh coriander.
2. Roll up and cut into 4 pieces. Wrap each piece with one slice of prosciutto; secure with a kitchen twine.
3. Place the wrapped chicken in a parchment-lined baking pan. Now, bake in the preheated oven at 385 degrees F for about 30 minutes.

Nutrition:
499 Calories
18.9g Fat
5.7g Carbs
41.6g Protein
0.6g Fiber

BOOZY GLAZED CHICKEN

Preparation Time: 40 minutes
Cooking Time: 1 hour + marinating time
Servings: 4
Ingredients:

- 2 pounds chicken drumettes
- 2 tablespoons ghee, at room temperature
- Sea salt and ground black pepper, to taste
- 1 teaspoon Mediterranean seasoning mix
- 2 vine-ripened tomatoes, pureed
- 3/4 cup rum
- 3 tablespoons coconut aminos
- A few drops of liquid Stevia
- 1 teaspoon chile peppers, minced
- 1 tablespoon minced fresh ginger
- 1 teaspoon ground cardamom

- 2 tablespoons fresh lemon juice, plus wedges for serving

Directions:

1. Toss the chicken with the melted ghee, salt, black pepper, and Mediterranean seasoning mix until well coated on all sides.
2. In another bowl, thoroughly combine the pureed tomato puree, rum, coconut aminos, Stevia, chile peppers, ginger, cardamom, and lemon juice.
3. Pour the tomato mixture over the chicken drumettes; let it marinate for 2 hours. Bake in the preheated oven at 410 degrees F for about 45 minutes.
4. Add in the reserved marinade and place under the preheated broiler for 10 minutes.

Nutrition:
307 Calories 12.1g Fat
2.7g Carbs
33.6g Protein
1.5g Fiber

FESTIVE TURKEY ROULADEN

Preparation Time: 15 minutes
Cooking Time: 30 minutes
Servings: 5
Ingredients:

- 2 pounds turkey fillet, marinated and cut into 10 pieces
- 10 strips prosciutto
- 1/2 teaspoon chili powder
- 1 teaspoon marjoram
- 1 sprig rosemary, finely chopped
- 2 tablespoons dry white wine
- 1 teaspoon garlic, finely minced
- 1 ½ tablespoons butter, room temperature
- 1 tablespoon Dijon mustard
- Sea salt and freshly ground black pepper, to your liking

Directions:

1. Start by preheating your oven to 430 degrees F.
2. Pat the turkey dry and cook in hot butter for about 3 minutes per side. Add in the mustard, chili powder, marjoram, rosemary, wine, and garlic.
3. Continue to cook for 2 minutes more. Wrap each turkey piece into one prosciutto strip and secure with toothpicks.
4. Roast in the preheated oven for about 30 minutes.

Nutrition:
286 Calories
9.7g Fat
6.9g Carbs
39.9g Protein
0.3g Fiber

PAN-FRIED CHORIZO SAUSAGE

Preparation Time: 10 minutes
Cooking Time: 20 minutes
Servings: 4
Ingredients:

- 16 ounces smoked turkey chorizo
- 1 ½ cups Asiago cheese, grated
- 1 teaspoon oregano
- 1 teaspoon basil
- 1 cup tomato puree

- 4 scallion stalks, chopped
- 1 teaspoon garlic paste
- Sea salt and ground black pepper, to taste
- 1 tablespoon dry sherry
- 1 tablespoon extra-virgin olive oil
- 2 tablespoons fresh coriander, roughly chopped

Directions:
1. Heat the oil in a frying pan over moderately high heat. Now, brown the turkey chorizo, crumbling with a fork for about 5 minutes.
2. Add in the other Ingredients, except for cheese; continue to cook for 10 minutes more or until cooked through.

Nutrition:
330 Calories
17.2g Fat
4.5g Carbs
34.4g Protein
1.6g Fiber

CHINESE BOK CHOY AND TURKEY SOUP

Preparation Time: 15 minutes
Cooking Time: 40 minutes
Servings: 8
Ingredients:
- 1/2 pound baby Bok choy, sliced into quarters lengthwise
- 2 pounds turkey carcass
- 1 tablespoon olive oil
- 1/2 cup leeks, chopped
- 1 celery rib, chopped
- 2 carrots, sliced
- 6 cups turkey stock
- Himalayan salt and black pepper, to taste

Directions:
1. In a heavy-bottomed pot, heat the olive oil until sizzling. Once hot, sauté the celery, carrots, leek and Bok choy for about 6 minutes.
2. Add the salt, pepper, turkey, and stock; bring to a boil.
3. Turn the heat to simmer. Continue to cook, partially covered, for about 35 minutes.

Nutrition:
211 Calories 11.8g Fat
3.1g Carbs
23.7g Protein
0.9g Fiber

HERBY CHICKEN MEATLOAF

Preparation Time: 20 minutes
Cooking Time: 30 minutes
Servings: 6
Ingredients:
- 2 ½ lb. ground chicken
- 3 tbsp flaxseed meal
- 2 large eggs
- 2 tbsp olive oil
- 1 lemon,1 tbsp juiced
- ¼ cup chopped parsley
- ¼ cup chopped oregano
- 4 garlic cloves, minced
- Lemon slices to garnish

Directions:
1. Preheat oven to 400 F. In a bowl, combine ground chicken and flaxseed meal; set aside. In a small bowl, whisk the eggs with olive oil, lemon juice, parsley, oregano, and garlic.
2. Pour the mixture onto the chicken mixture and mix well. Spoon into a greased loaf pan and press to fit. Bake for 40 minutes.
3. Remove the pan, drain the liquid, and let cool a bit. Slice, garnish with lemon slices, and serve.

Nutrition:
Cal 362
Net Carbs 1.3g
Fat 24g
Protein 35g

LOVELY PULLED CHICKEN EGG BITES

Preparation Time: 15 minutes
Cooking Time: 30 minutes
Servings: 4
Ingredients:
- 2 tbsp butter
- 1 chicken breast
- 2 tbsp chopped green onions
- ½ tsp red chili flakes
- 12 eggs
- ¼ cup grated Monterey Jack

Directions:
1. Preheat oven to 400 F. Line a 12-hole muffin tin with cupcake liners. Melt butter in a skillet over medium heat and cook the chicken until brown on each side, 10 minutes.
2. Transfer to a plate and shred with 2 forks. Divide between muffin holes along with green onions and red chili flakes.
3. Crack an egg into each muffin hole and scatter the cheese on top. Bake for 15 minutes until eggs set. Serve.

Nutrition:
Cal 393
Net Carbs 0.5g
Fat 27g
Protein 34g

CREAMY MUSTARD CHICKEN WITH SHIRATAKI

Preparation Time: 20 minutes
Cooking Time: 30 minutes
Servings: 4
Ingredients:
- 2 (8 oz.) packs angel hair shirataki
- 4 chicken breasts, cut into strips
- 1 cup chopped mustard greens
- 1 yellow bell pepper, sliced
- 1 tbsp olive oil
- 1 yellow onion, finely sliced
- 1 garlic clove, minced
- 1 tbsp wholegrain mustard
- 5 tbsp heavy cream
- 1 tbsp chopped parsley

Directions:

1. Boil 2 cups of water in a medium pot.
2. Strain the shirataki pasta and rinse well under hot running water. Allow proper draining and pour the shirataki pasta into the boiling water.
3. Cook for 3 minutes and strain again. Place a dry skillet and stir-fry the shirataki pasta until visibly dry, 1-2 minutes; set aside.
4. Heat olive oil in a skillet, season the chicken with salt and pepper and cook for 8-10 minutes; set aside. Stir in onion, bell pepper, and garlic and cook until softened, 5 minutes.
5. Mix in mustard and heavy cream; simmer for 2 minutes and mix in the chicken and mustard greens for 2 minutes. Stir in shirataki pasta, garnish with parsley and serve.

Nutrition:

Cal 692
Net Carbs 15g
Fats 38g
Protein 65g

CHAPTER 16:

BEEF RECIPES

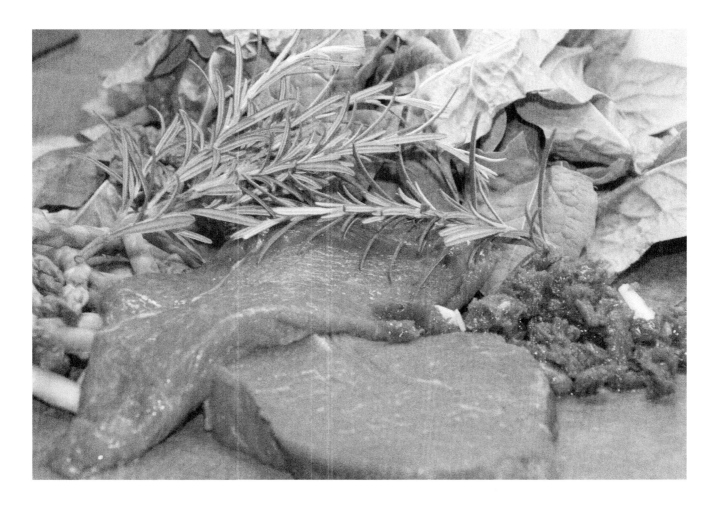

MUSTARD-LEMON BEEF

Preparation Time: 15 minutes
Cooking Time: 25 minutes
Servings: 4
Ingredients:

- 2 tbsp olive oil
- 1 tbsp fresh rosemary, chopped
- 2 garlic cloves, minced
- 1 ½ lb. beef rump steak, thinly sliced
- Salt and black pepper to taste
- 1 shallot, chopped
- ½ cup heavy cream
- ½ cup beef stock
- 1 tbsp mustard
- 2 tsp Worcestershire sauce
- 2 tsp lemon juice
- 1 tsp erythritol - 2 tbsp butter
- 1 tbsp fresh rosemary, chopped
- 1 tbsp fresh thyme, chopped

Directions:

1. In a bowl, combine 1 tbsp of oil with black pepper, garlic, rosemary, and salt. Toss in the beef to coat and set aside for some minutes. Heat a pan with the rest of the oil over medium heat, place in the beef steak, and cook for 6 minutes, flipping halfway through. Set aside and keep warm.
2. Melt the butter in the pan. Add in the shallot and cook for 3 minutes. Stir in the stock, Worcestershire sauce, erythritol, thyme, cream, mustard, and rosemary and cook for 8 minutes. Mix in the lemon juice, pepper, and salt. Arrange the beef slices on serving plates, sprinkle over the sauce, and enjoy!

Nutrition: Kcal 435 Fat 30g Net Carbs 5g Protein 32g

RIBEYE STEAK WITH SHITAKE MUSHROOMS

Preparation Time: 10 minutes
Cooking Time: 25 minutes
Servings: 4
Ingredients:

- 1 lb. ribeye steaks
- 1 tbsp butter
- 2 tbsp olive oil
- 1 cup shitake mushrooms, sliced
- Salt and black pepper to taste
- 2 tbsp fresh parsley, chopped

Directions:

1. Heat the olive oil in a pan over medium heat. Rub the steaks with salt and black pepper and cook about 4 minutes per side; reserve.
2. Melt the butter in the pan and cook the shitakes for 4 minutes. Scatter the parsley over and pour the mixture over the steaks to serve.

Nutrition:
Calories: 406 Fat: 21g Carb: 11g, Protein: 10g

PARSLEY BEEF BURGERS

Preparation Time: 10 minutes
Cooking Time: 25 minutes
Servings: 6
Ingredients:

- 2 lb. ground beef

- 1 tbsp onion flakes
- ¾ cup almond flour
- ¼ cup beef broth
- 2 tbsp fresh parsley, chopped
- 1 tbsp Worcestershire sauce

Directions:

1. Combine all ingredients in a bowl. Mix well with your hands and make 6 patties out of the mixture. Arrange on a lined baking sheet. Bake at 370ºF for about 18 minutes, until nice and crispy. Serve.

Nutrition:
Kcal 354
Fat: 28g
Net Carbs: 2.5g
Protein: 27g

BEEF CAULIFLOWER CURRY

Preparation Time: 15 minutes
Cooking Time: 26 minutes
Servings: 6
Ingredients:

- 1 tbsp olive oil
- 1 ½ lb. ground beef
- 1 tbsp ginger paste
- 1 tsp garam masala
- 1 (7 oz.) can whole tomatoes
- 1 head cauliflower, cut into florets
- Salt to taste
- 2 garlic cloves, minced
- ½ tsp hot paprika

Directions:

2. Heat oil in a saucepan over medium heat. Add the beef, ginger, garlic, garam masala, paprika, and salt and cook for 5 minutes while breaking any lumps. Stir in the tomatoes and cauliflower. Cook covered for 6 minutes.
3. Add ½ cup water and bring to a boil. Simmer for 10 minutes or until the water has reduced by half. Spoon the curry into serving bowls and serve with shirataki rice.

Nutrition:
Kcal 374
Fat 33g
Net Carbs 2g
Protein 22g

ITALIAN BEEF RAGOUT

Preparation Time: 40 minutes
Cooking Time: 1 hour 55 minutes
Servings: 4
Ingredients:

- 1 lb. chuck steak, cubed
- 2 tbsp olive oil
- Salt and black pepper to taste
- 2 tbsp almond flour
- 1 onion, diced
- ½ cup dry white wine
- 1 red bell pepper, seeded and diced
- 2 tsp Worcestershire sauce
- 4 oz. tomato puree
- 3 tsp smoked paprika
- 1 cup beef broth
- 2 tbsp fresh thyme, chopped

Directions:

1. Lightly dredge the meat in the almond flour. Place a large skillet over medium heat, add the olive oil to heat and then sauté the onion and bell pepper for 3 minutes. Stir in paprika.
2. Add the beef and cook for 10 minutes in total while turning them halfway. Stir in white wine and let it reduce by half, about 3 minutes.
3. Add in Worcestershire sauce, tomato puree, beef broth, salt, and pepper. Let the mixture boil for 2 minutes, reduce the heat, and let simmer for 1 ½ hours, stirring often. Serve garnished with thyme.

Nutrition:
Calories: 129.2
Fat: 4.7g
Carb: 16.3g,
Protein: 27g

BEEF MEATBALLS

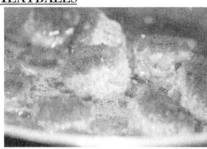

Preparation Time: 23 minutes
Cooking Time: 35 minutes
Servings: 4
Ingredients:

- ½ cup pork rinds, crushed
- 1 egg
- Salt and black pepper to taste
- 1 ½ lb. ground beef
- 10 oz. canned onion soup
- 1 tbsp almond flour
- ¼ cup free-sugar ketchup
- 3 tsp Worcestershire sauce
- ½ tsp dry mustard

Directions:

1. In a bowl, combine 1/3 cup of the onion soup with the beef, pepper, pork rinds, egg, and salt. Shape the mixture into 12 meatballs. Heat a greased pan over medium heat. Brown the meatballs for 12 minutes.
2. In a separate bowl, combine the rest of the soup with the almond flour, dry mustard, ketchup, Worcestershire sauce, and ¼ cup water. Pour this over the beef meatballs, cover the pan, and cook for 10 minutes as you stir occasionally. Split among bowls and serve.

Nutrition:
Kcal 332 Fat 18g
Net Carbs 7g Protein 25g

BEEF & ALE POT ROAST

Preparation Time: 30 minutes
Cooking Time: 2 hours 20 minutes
Servings: 6
Ingredients:

- 1 ½ lb. brisket

- 2 tbsp olive oil
- 8 baby carrots, peeled
- 2 medium red onions, quartered
- 1 celery stalk, cut into chunks
- Salt and black pepper to taste
- 2 bay leaves
- 1 ½ cups low carb beer (ale)

Directions:

1. Preheat oven to 370ºF. Heat the olive oil in a large skillet over medium heat. Season the brisket with salt and pepper.
2. Brown the meat on both sides for 8 minutes. After, transfer to a deep casserole dish. In the dish, arrange the carrots, onions, celery, and bay leaves around the brisket and pour the beer all over it.
3. Cover the pot and cook in the oven for 2 hours. When ready, remove the casserole. Transfer the beef to a chopping board and cut it into thick slices. Serve the beef and vegetables with a drizzle of the sauce.

Nutrition:
Calories: 302.2
Fat: 22.7g
Carb: 9.3g,
Protein: 8g

BEEF TRIPE POT

Preparation Time: 10 minutes
Cooking Time: 1 hour 30 minutes
Servings: 6
Ingredients:

- 1 ½ lb. beef tripe, cleaned
- 4 cups buttermilk
- Salt and black pepper to taste
- 3 tbsp olive oil
- 2 onions, sliced
- 4 garlic cloves, minced
- 3 tomatoes, diced
- 1 tsp paprika
- 2 chili peppers, minced

Directions:

1. Put the tripe in a bowl and cover with buttermilk. Refrigerate for 3 hours to extract bitterness and gamey taste.
2. Remove from buttermilk, drain and rinse well under cold running water. Place in a pot over medium heat and cover with water. Bring to a boil and cook about for 1 hour until tender. Remove the tripe with a perforated spoon and let cool. Strain the broth and reserve. Chop the cooled tripe.
3. Heat the oil in a skillet over medium heat. Sauté the onions, garlic, and chili peppers for 3 minutes until soft. Stir in the paprika and add in the tripe. Cook for 5-6 minutes. Include the tomatoes and 4 cups of the reserved tripe broth and cook for 10 minutes. Adjust the seasoning with salt and pepper. Serve.

Nutrition:
Kcal 248
Fat 12.8g
Net Carbs 4g
Protein 8g

BEEF STOVIES

Preparation Time: 12 minutes
Cooking Time: 45 minutes
Servings: 4
Ingredients:

- 1 lb. ground beef
- 1 large onion, chopped
- 2 parsnips, peeled and chopped
- 1 large carrot, chopped
- 2 tbsp olive oil
- 2 garlic cloves, minced
- Salt and black pepper to taste
- 1 cup chicken broth
- ¼ tsp allspice
- 2 tsp fresh rosemary, chopped
- 1 tbsp Worcestershire sauce
- ½ small cabbage, shredded

Directions:

1. Heat the olive oil in a skillet over medium heat and cook the beef for 4 minutes. Season with salt and pepper, stirring occasionally while breaking the lumps in it.
2. Add in onion, garlic, carrot, rosemary, and parsnips.
3. Stir and cook for a minute, and pour in the chicken broth, allspice, and Worcestershire sauce.
4. Reduce the heat to low and cook for 20 minutes. Stir in the cabbage, season with salt and black pepper, and cook further for 15 minutes. Turn the heat off, plate the stovies, and serve warm.

Nutrition:
Kcal 316
Fat 18g
Net Carbs 3g
Protein 14g

BEEF AND SAUSAGE MEDLEY

Preparation Time: 10 minutes
Cooking Time: 27 minutes
Servings: 8
Ingredients:

- 1 teaspoon butter
- 2 beef sausages, casing removed and sliced
- 2 pounds (907 g) beef steak, cubed
- 1 yellow onion, sliced
- 2 fresh ripe tomatoes, puréed
- 1 jalapeño pepper, chopped
- 1 red bell pepper, chopped
- 1½ cups roasted vegetable broth
- 2 cloves garlic, minced
- 1 teaspoon Old Bay seasoning
- 2 bay leaves
- 1 sprig thyme
- 1 sprig rosemary
- ½ teaspoon paprika
- Sea salt and ground black pepper, to taste

Directions:

1. Press the Sauté button to heat up the Instant Pot. Melt the butter and cook the sausage and steak for 4 minutes, stirring periodically. Set aside.
2. Add the onion and sauté for 3 minutes or until softened and translucent. Add the remaining ingredients, including reserved beef and sausage.
3. Secure the lid. Choose Manual mode and set time for 20 minutes on High Pressure.
4. Once cooking is complete, use a quick pressure release. Carefully remove the lid.
5. Serve immediately.

Nutrition:
Calories: 319
Fat: 14.0g
Protein: 42.8g
Carbs: 6.3g
Net carbs: 1.8g
Fiber: 4.5g

BEEF BACK RIBS WITH BARBECUE GLAZE

Preparation Time: 10 minutes
Cooking Time: 35 minutes
Servings: 4
Ingredients:

- ½ cup water
- 1 (3-pound / 1.4-kg) rack beef back ribs, prepared with rub of choice
- ¼ cup unsweetened tomato purée
- ¼ teaspoon Worcestershire sauce
- ¼ teaspoon garlic powder
- 2 teaspoons apple cider vinegar
- ¼ teaspoon liquid smoke
- ¼ teaspoon smoked paprika
- 3 tablespoons Swerve
- Dash of cayenne pepper

Directions:

1. Pour the water in the pot and place the trivet inside.
2. Arrange the ribs on top of the trivet.
3. Close the lid. Select Manual mode and set cooking time for 25 minutes on High Pressure.
4. Meanwhile, prepare the glaze by whisking together the tomato purée, Worcestershire sauce, garlic powder, vinegar, liquid smoke, paprika, Swerve, and cayenne in a medium bowl. Heat the broiler.
5. When timer beeps, quick release the pressure. Open the lid. Remove the ribs and place on a baking sheet.
6. Brush a layer of glaze on the ribs. Put under the broiler for 5 minutes.
7. Remove from the broiler and brush with glaze again. Put back under the broiler for 5 more minutes, or until the tops are sticky.
8. Serve immediately.

Nutrition:
Calories: 758
Fat: 26.8g
Protein: 33.7g
Carbs: 0.9g
Net carbs: 0.7g
Fiber: 0.2g

BEEF BIG MAC SALAD

Preparation Time: 10 minutes
Cooking Time: 9 minutes
Servings: 2
Ingredients:

- 5 ounces (142 g) ground beef
- 1 teaspoon ground black pepper
- 1 tablespoon sesame oil
- 1 cup lettuce, chopped
- ¼ cup Monterey Jack cheese, shredded
- 2 ounces (57 g) dill pickles, sliced
- 1 ounce (28 g) scallions, chopped
- 1 tablespoon heavy cream

Directions:

1. In a mixing bowl, combine the ground beef and ground black pepper. Shape the mixture into mini burgers.
2. Pour the sesame oil in the Instant Pot and heat for 3 minutes on Sauté mode.
3. Place the mini hamburgers in the hot oil and cook for 3 minutes on each side.
4. Meanwhile, in a salad bowl, mix the chopped lettuce, shredded cheese, dill pickles, scallions, and heavy cream. Toss to mix well.
5. Top the salad with cooked mini burgers. Serve immediately.

Nutrition:
Calories: 284
Fat: 18.5g
Protein: 25.7g
Carbs: 3.5g
Net carbs: 2.3g
Fiber: 1.2g

BEEF BOURGUIGNON

Preparation Time: 15 minutes
Cooking Time: 35 minutes
Servings: 6
Ingredients:

- 3 ounces (85 g) bacon, chopped
- 1 pound (454 g) beef tenderloin, chopped
- ¼ cup apple cider vinegar
- ¼ teaspoon ground coriander
- ¼ teaspoon xanthan gum
- 1 teaspoon dried oregano
- 1 teaspoon unsweetened tomato purée
- 1 cup beef broth

Directions:

1. Put the bacon in the Instant Pot and cook for 5 minutes on Sauté mode. Flip the bacon with a spatula every 1 minute.
2. Add the chopped beef tenderloin, apple cider vinegar, ground coriander, xanthan gum, and dried oregano.
3. Add the tomato purée and beef broth. Stir to mix well and close the lid.
4. Select Manual mode and set cooking time for 30 minutes on High Pressure.
5. When timer beeps, make a quick pressure release. Open the lid.
6. Serve immediately.

Nutrition:
Calories: 245
Fat: 13.1g
Protein: 28.0g
Carbs: 1.3g
Net carbs: 0.6g
Fiber: 0.7g

BEEF BRISKET WITH CABBAGE

Preparation Time: 15 minutes
Cooking Time: 1 hour 7 minutes
Servings: 8
Ingredients:

- 3 pounds (1.4 kg) corned beef brisket
- 4 cups water
- 3 garlic cloves, minced
- 2 teaspoons yellow mustard seed
- 2 teaspoons black peppercorns
- 3 celery stalks, chopped
- ½ large white onion, chopped
- 1 green cabbage, cut into quarters

Directions:

1. Add the brisket to the Instant Pot. Pour the water into the pot. Add the garlic, mustard seed, and black peppercorns.
2. Lock the lid. Select Meat/Stew mode and set cooking time for 50 minutes on High Pressure.
3. When cooking is complete, allow the pressure to release naturally for 20 minutes, then release any remaining pressure. Open the lid and transfer only the brisket to a platter.
4. Add the celery, onion, and cabbage to the pot.
5. Lock the lid. Select Soup mode and set cooking time for 12 minutes on High Pressure.
6. When cooking is complete, quick release the pressure. Open the lid, add the brisket back to the pot and let warm in the pot for 5 minutes.
7. Transfer the warmed brisket back to the platter and thinly slice. Transfer the vegetables to the platter. Serve hot.

Nutrition:
Calories: 357 Fat: 25.5g
Protein: 26.3g Carbs: 7.3g
Net carbs: 5.3g Fiber: 2.0g

BEEF CARNE GUISADA

Preparation Time: 10 minutes
Cooking Time: 20 minutes
Servings: 4
Ingredients:

- 2 tomatoes, chopped
- 1 red bell pepper, chopped
- ½ onion, chopped
- 3 garlic cloves, chopped
- 1 teaspoon ancho chili powder
- 1 tablespoon ground cumin
- ½ teaspoon dried oregano
- 1 teaspoons salt
- 1 teaspoon freshly ground black pepper
- 1 teaspoon smoked paprika
- 1 pound (454 g) beef chuck, cut into large pieces

- ¾ cup water, plus 2 tablespoons
- ¼ teaspoon xanthan gum

Directions:

1. In a blender, purée the tomatoes, bell pepper, onion, garlic, chili powder, cumin, oregano, salt, pepper, and paprika.
2. Put the beef pieces in the Instant Pot. Pour in the blended mixture.
3. Use ¾ cup of water to wash out the blender and pour the liquid into the pot.
4. Lock the lid. Select Manual mode and set cooking time for 20 minutes on High Pressure.
5. When cooking is complete, quick release the pressure. Unlock the lid.
6. Switch the pot to Sauté mode. Bring the stew to a boil.
7. Put the xanthan gum and 2 tablespoons of water into the boiling stew and stir until it thickens.
8. Serve immediately.

Nutrition:

Calories: 326 Fat: 22.0g
Protein: 23.0g Carbs: 9.0g
Net carbs: 7.0g Fiber: 2.0g

CHAPTER 17:

PORK RECIPES

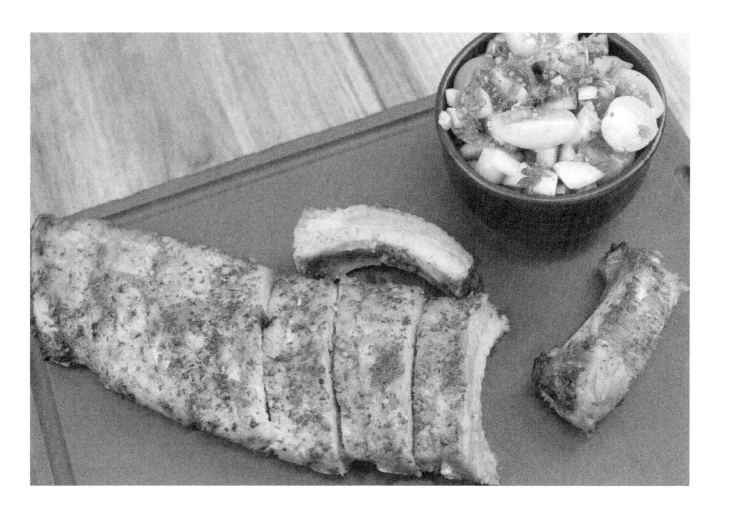

CILANTRO GARLIC PORK CHOPS

Preparation Time: 10 Minutes
Cooking Time: 15 Minutes
Servings: 4
Ingredients:

- 1 pound boneless center-cut pork chops, pounded to ¼ inch thick
- Sea salt, for seasoning
- Freshly ground black pepper, for seasoning
- ¼ cup good-quality olive oil, divided
- ¼ cup finely chopped fresh cilantro
- 1 tablespoon minced garlic
- Juice of 1 lime

Directions:

1. Marinate the pork. Pat the pork chops dry and season them lightly with salt and pepper. Place them in a large bowl, add 2 tablespoons of the olive oil, and the cilantro, garlic, and lime juice. Toss to coat the chops. Cover the bowl and marinate the chops at room temperature for 30 minutes.
   Cook the pork. In a large skillet over medium-high heat, warm the remaining 2 tablespoons of olive oil. Add the pork chops in a single layer and fry them, turning them once, until they're just cooked through and still juicy, 6 to 7 minutes per side.
2.
   Serve. Divide the chops between four plates and serve them immediately.

Nutrition:
Calories: 249
Total fat: 16g
Total carbs: 2g
Fiber: 0g;
Net carbs: 2g
Sodium: 261mg
Protein: 25g

SPINACH FETA STUFFED PORK

Preparation Time: 15 Minutes
Cooking Time: 30 Minutes
Servings: 4
Ingredients:

- 4 ounces crumbled feta cheese
- ¾ cup chopped frozen spinach, thawed and liquid squeezed out
- 3 tablespoons chopped Kalamata olives
- 4 (4-ounce) center pork chops, 2 inches thick
- Sea salt, for seasoning
- Freshly ground black pepper, for seasoning
- 3 tablespoons good-quality olive oil

Directions:

1. Preheat the oven. Set the oven temperature to 400°F.
2. Make the filling. In a small bowl, mix together the feta, spinach, and olives until everything is well combined.
3. Stuff the pork chops. Make a horizontal slit in the side of each chop to create a pocket, making sure you don't cut all the way through. Stuff the filling equally between the chops and secure the slits with toothpicks. Lightly season the stuffed chops with salt and pepper.
4. Brown the chops. In a large oven-safe skillet over medium-high heat, warm the olive oil.

5. Add the chops and sear them until they're browned all over, about 10 minutes in total.
6. Roast the chops. Place the skillet in the oven and roast the chops for 20 minutes or until they're cooked through.
7. Serve. Let the meat rest for 10 minutes and then remove the toothpicks. Divide the pork chops between four plates and serve them immediately.

Nutrition:
Calories: 342
Total fat: 24g
Total carbs: 3g
Fiber: 1g;
Net carbs: 2g
Sodium: 572mg
Protein: 28g

COCONUT MILK GINGER MARINATED PORK TENDERLOIN

Preparation Time: 5 Minutes
Cooking Time: 25 Minutes
Servings: 4
Ingredients:

- ¼ cup coconut oil, divided
- 1½ pounds boneless pork chops, about ¾ inch thick
- 1 tablespoon grated fresh ginger
- 2 teaspoons minced garlic
- 1 cup coconut milk
- 1 teaspoon chopped fresh basil
- Juice of 1 lime
- ½ cup shredded unsweetened coconut

Directions:

1. Brown the pork. In a large skillet over medium heat, warm 2 tablespoons of the coconut oil. Add the pork chops to the skillet and brown them all over, turning them several times, about 10 minutes in total.
2. Braise the pork. Move the pork to the side of the skillet and add the remaining 2 tablespoons of coconut oil. Add the ginger and garlic and sauté until they've softened, about 2 minutes. Stir in the coconut milk, basil, and lime juice and move the pork back to the center of the skillet. Cover the skillet and simmer until the pork is just cooked through and very tender, 12 to 15 minutes.
3. Serve. Divide the pork chops between four plates and top them with the shredded coconut.

Nutrition:
Calories: 479
Total fat: 38g
Total carbs: 6g
Fiber: 3g;
Net carbs: 3g
Sodium: 318mg
Protein: 32g

GRILLED PORK CHOPS WITH GREEK SALSA

Preparation Time: 15 Minutes
Cooking Time: 15 Minutes
Servings: 4
Ingredients:

- ¼ cup good-quality olive oil, divided
- 1 tablespoon red wine vinegar

- 3 teaspoons chopped fresh oregano, divided
- 1 teaspoon minced garlic
- 4 (4-ounce) boneless center-cut loin pork chops
- ½ cup halved cherry tomatoes
- ½ yellow bell pepper, diced
- ½ English cucumber, chopped
- ¼ red onion, chopped
- 1 tablespoon balsamic vinegar
- Sea salt, for seasoning
- Freshly ground black pepper, for seasoning

Directions:

1. Marinate the pork. In a medium bowl, stir together 3 tablespoons of the olive oil, the vinegar, 2 teaspoons of the oregano, and the garlic. Add the pork chops to the bowl, turning them to get them coated with the marinade. Cover the bowl and place it in the refrigerator for 30 minutes.
2. Make the salsa. While the pork is marinating, in a medium bowl, stir together the remaining 1 tablespoon of olive oil, the tomatoes, yellow bell pepper, cucumber, red onion, vinegar, and the remaining 1 teaspoon of oregano. Season the salsa with salt and pepper. Set the bowl aside.
3. Grill the pork chops. Heat a grill to medium-high heat. Remove the pork chops from the marinade and grill them until just cooked through, 6 to 8 minutes per side.
4. Serve. Rest the pork for 5 minutes. Divide the pork between four plates and serve them with a generous scoop of the salsa.

Nutrition:
Calories: 277
Total fat: 19g
Total carbs: 4g
Fiber: 1g;
Net carbs: 3g
Sodium: 257mg; Protein: 25g

GRILLED HERBED PORK KEBABS

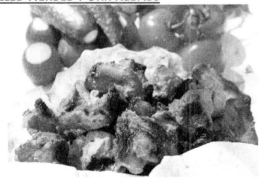

Preparation Time: 10 Minutes
Cooking Time: 15 Minutes
Servings: 4
Ingredients:

- ¼ cup good-quality olive oil
- 1 tablespoon minced garlic
- 2 teaspoons dried oregano
- 1 teaspoon dried basil
- 1 teaspoon dried parsley
- ½ teaspoon sea salt
- 1/4 teaspoon freshly ground black pepper
- 1 (1-pound) pork tenderloin, cut into 1½-inch pieces

Directions:

1. Marinate the pork. In a medium bowl, stir together the olive oil, garlic, oregano, basil, parsley, salt, and pepper. Add the pork pieces and toss to coat them in the marinade. Cover the bowl and place it in the refrigerator for 2 to 4 hours.
2. Make the kebabs. Divide the pork pieces between four skewers, making sure not to crowd the meat.
3. Grill the kebabs. Preheat your grill to medium-high heat. Grill the skewers for about 12 minutes, turning to cook all sides of the pork, until the pork is cooked through.
4. Serve. Rest the skewers for 5 minutes. Divide the skewers between four plates and serve them immediately.

Nutrition:
Calories: 261
Total fat: 18g
Total carbs: 1g
Fiber: 0g;
Net carbs: 1g
Sodium: 60mg
Protein: 24

ITALIAN SAUSAGE BROCCOLI SAUTÉ

Preparation Time: 10 Minutes
Cooking Time: 20 Minutes
Servings: 4
Ingredients:

- 2 tablespoons good-quality olive oil
- 1 pound Italian sausage meat, hot or mild
- 4 cups small broccoli florets
- 1 tablespoon minced garlic
- Freshly ground black pepper, for seasoning

Directions:

1. Cook the sausage. In a large skillet over medium heat, warm the olive oil. Add the sausage and sauté it until it's cooked through, 8 to 10 minutes. Transfer the sausage to a plate with a slotted spoon and set the plate aside.
2. Sauté the vegetables. Add the broccoli to the skillet and sauté it until its tender, about 6 minutes. Stir in the garlic and sauté for another 3 minutes.
3. Finish the dish. Return the sausage to the skillet and toss to combine it with the other ingredients. Season the mixture with pepper.
4. Serve. Divide the mixture between four plates and serve it immediately.

Nutrition:
Calories: 486 Total fat: 43g
Total carbs: 7g Fiber: 2g;
Net carbs: 5g Sodium: 513mg
Protein: 19g

CLASSIC SAUSAGE AND PEPPERS

Preparation Time: 10 Minutes
Cooking Time: 35 Minutes
Servings: 6
Ingredients:

- 1½ pounds sweet Italian sausages (or hot if you prefer)
- 2 tablespoons good-quality olive oil
- 1 red bell pepper, cut into thin strips
- 1 yellow bell pepper, cut into thin strips

- 1 orange bell pepper, cut into thin strips
- 1 red onion, thinly sliced
- 1 tablespoon minced garlic
- ½ cup white wine
- Sea salt, for seasoning
- Freshly ground black pepper, for seasoning

Directions:

1. Cook the sausage. Preheat a grill to medium-high and grill the sausages, turning them several times, until they're cooked through, about 12 minutes in total. Let the sausages rest for 15 minutes and then cut them into 2-inch pieces.
2. Sauté the vegetables. In a large skillet over medium-high heat, warm the olive oil. Add the red, yellow, and orange bell peppers, and the red onion and garlic and sauté until they're tender, about 10 minutes.
3. Finish the dish. Add the sausage to the skillet along with the white wine and sauté for 10 minutes.
4. Serve. Divide the mixture between four plates, season it with salt and pepper, and serve.

Nutrition:
Calories: 450
Total fat: 40g
Total carbs: 5g
Fiber: 1g;
Net carbs: 4g
Sodium: 554mg
Protein: 17g

LEMON-INFUSED PORK RIB ROAST

Preparation Time: 10 Minutes
Cooking Time: 1 Hour
Servings: 6
Ingredients:

- ¼ cup good-quality olive oil
- Zest and juice of 1 lemon
- Zest and juice of 1 orange
- 4 rosemary sprigs, lightly crushed
- 4 thyme sprigs, lightly crushed
- 1 (4-bone) pork rib roast, about 2½ pounds
- 6 garlic cloves, peeled
- Sea salt, for seasoning
- Freshly ground black pepper, for seasoning

Directions:

1. Make the marinade. In a large bowl, combine the olive oil, lemon zest, lemon juice, orange zest, orange juice, rosemary sprigs, and thyme sprigs.
2. Marinate the roast. Use a small knife to make six 1-inch-deep slits in the fatty side of the roast. Stuff the garlic cloves in the slits. Put the roast in the bowl with the marinade and turn it to coat it well with the marinade. Cover the bowl and refrigerate it overnight, turning the roast in the marinade several times.
3. Preheat the oven. Set the oven temperature to 350°F.
4. Roast the pork. Remove the pork from the marinade and season it with salt and pepper, then put it in a baking dish and let it come to room temperature. Roast the pork until it's cooked through (145°F to 160°F internal

temperature), about 1 hour. Throw out any leftover marinade.
5. Serve. Let the pork rest for 10 minutes, then cut it into slices and arrange the slices on a platter. Serve it warm.

Nutrition:
Calories: 403
Total fat: 30g
Total carbs: 1g
Fiber: 0g;
Net carbs: 1g
Sodium: 113mg
Protein: 30g

PORK MEATBALL PARMESAN

Preparation Time: 15 Minutes
Cooking Time: 30 Minutes
Servings: 6
Ingredients:
For The Meatballs:

- 1¼ Pounds ground pork
- ½ cup almond flour
- ½ cup Parmesan cheese
- 1 egg, lightly beaten
- 1 tablespoon chopped fresh parsley
- 1 teaspoon minced garlic
- 1 teaspoon chopped fresh oregano
- ¼ teaspoon sea salt
- 1/8 teaspoon freshly ground black pepper
- 2 tablespoons good-quality olive oil

FOR THE PARMIGIANA:

- 1 cup sugar-free tomato sauce
- 1 cup shredded mozzarella cheese

Directions:

1. Make the meatballs. In a large bowl, mix together the ground pork, almond flour, Parmesan, egg, parsley, garlic, oregano, salt, and pepper until everything is well mixed. Roll the pork mixture into 1½-inch meatballs.
2. Cook the meatballs. In a large skillet over medium-high heat, warm the olive oil. Add the meatballs to the skillet and cook them, turning them several times, until they're thoroughly cooked through, about 15 minutes in total.

TO MAKE THE PARMIGIANA:

3. Preheat the oven. Set the oven temperature to 350°F.
4. Assemble the parmigiana. Transfer the meatballs to a 9-by-9-inch baking dish and top them with the tomato sauce. Sprinkle with the mozzarella and bake for 15 minutes or until the cheese is melted and golden.
5. Serve. Divide the meatballs and sauce between six bowls and serve it immediately.

Nutrition:
Calories: 403
Total fat: 32g
Total carbs: 1g
Fiber: 0g;
Net carbs: 1g
Sodium: 351mg
Protein: 25g

CHAPTER 18:

LAMB RECIPES

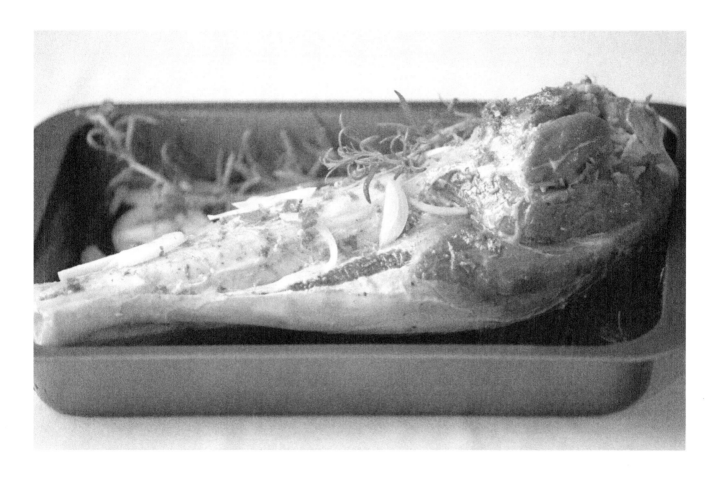

CHIPOTLE LAMB RIBS

Preparation Time: 15 minutes
Cooking Time: 20 minutes
Servings: 6
Ingredients:

- 2-pound lamb ribs
- 1 tablespoon chipotle pepper, minced
- 2 tablespoons sesame oil
- 1 teaspoon apple cider vinegar

Directions:

1. Mix lamb ribs with all ingredients and leave to marinate for 10 minutes.
2. Then transfer the lamb ribs and all marinade in the baking tray and cook the meat in the oven at 360F for 40 minutes. Flip the ribs on another side after 20 minutes of cooking.

Nutrition:
Calories 392 Fat 24.7
Fiber 0
Carbs 0.2
Protein 39.6

LAMB AND PECAN SALAD

Preparation Time: 10 minutes
Cooking Time: 10 minutes
Servings: 4
Ingredients:

- 2 lamb chops
- 1 tablespoon sesame oil
- 2 pecans, chopped
- 2 cups lettuce, chopped
- 1 teaspoon cayenne pepper
- 1 tablespoon avocado oil

Directions:

1. Sprinkle the lamb chops with cayenne pepper and put in the hot skillet.
2. Add sesame oil and roast the meat for 4 minutes per side.
3. Then chops the lamb chops and put them in the salad bowl.
4. Add all remaining ingredients and carefully mix the salad.

Nutrition:
Calories 168
Fat 12.1
Fiber 1
Carbs 2.3
Protein 12.9

HOT SAUCE LAMB

Preparation Time: 10 minutes
Cooking Time: 35 minutes
Servings: 4
Ingredients:

- 2 teaspoons paprika
- 1-pound lamb fillet, chopped
- 1 tablespoon coconut oil
- 4 tablespoons keto hot sauce
- ½ cup of water

Directions:

1. Pour water in the saucepan and bring it to boil.

2. Add lamb and boil it for 20 minutes.
3. After this, preheat the skillet well.
4. Add boiled lamb fillet, coconut oil, and paprika.
5. Roast the ingredients for 6 minutes per side or until the meat is light brown.
6. Then add hot sauce and carefully mix the meal.

Nutrition:
Calories 245
Fat 11.9
Fiber 0.4
Carbs 0.8
Protein 32.1

MUSTARD LAMB CHOPS

Preparation Time: 10 minutes
Cooking Time: 40 minutes
Servings: 4
Ingredients:

- 1 cup spinach
- 3 tablespoons mustard
- 2 tablespoons sesame oil
- ½ teaspoon ground turmeric
- 4 lamb chops

Directions:

1. Blend the spinach and mix it with mustard, sesame oil, and ground turmeric.
2. Then rub the lamb chops with the mustard mixture and put in the baking pan.
3. Bake the meat at 355F for 40 minutes. Flip the meat after 20 minutes of cooking.

Nutrition:
Calories 102
Fat 9.3
Fiber 1.5
Carbs 3.4
Protein 2.3

GINGER LAMB CHOPS

Preparation Time: 15 minutes
Cooking Time: 30 minutes
Servings: 6
Ingredients:

- 6 lamb chops
- 1 tablespoon keto tomato paste
- 1 teaspoon minced ginger
- 2 tablespoons avocado oil
- 1 teaspoon plain yogurt

Directions:

1. Mix plain yogurt with keto tomato paste and minced ginger.
2. Then put the lamb chops in the yogurt mixture and marinate for 10-15 minutes.
3. After this, transfer the mixture in the tray, add avocado oil, and cook the meat at 360F in the oven for 30 minutes.

Nutrition:
Calories 330
Fat 26.6
Fiber 0.4
Carbs 1
Protein 19.3

PARMESAN LAMB

Preparation Time: 10 minutes
Cooking Time: 20 minutes
Servings: 4
Ingredients:

- 4 lamb chops
- 2 oz. Parmesan, grated
- ½ cup plain yogurt
- 3 scallions, sliced
- 1 tablespoon butter, softened

Directions:

1. Melt the butter in the saucepan. Add scallions and roast it for 3-4 minutes.
2. Then stir the scallions and add lamb chops.
3. Roast them for 2 minutes per side.
4. Add yogurt and close the lid. Cook the meat for 10 minutes.
5. After this, top the meat with Parmesan and cook it for 2 minutes more.

Nutrition:
Calories 262
Fat 12.6
Fiber 0.6
Carbs 5.2
Protein 30.5

CLOVE LAMB

Preparation Time: 10 minutes
Cooking Time: 25 minutes
Servings: 4
Ingredients:

- 1 teaspoon ground clove
- 2 tablespoons butter
- 1 teaspoon ground paprika
- 1 teaspoon dried rosemary
- ¼ cup of water
- 12 oz. lamb fillet

Directions:

1. In the shallow bowl, mix ground clove with ground paprika, and dried rosemary.
2. Rub the lamb fillet with spices and grease with butter.
3. Then put the meat in the hot skillet and roast it for 5 minutes per side on the low heat.
4. Add water. Close the lid and cook the lamb on medium heat for 15 minutes.

Nutrition:
Calories 55
Fat 6
Fiber 0.5
Carbs 0.8
Protein 0.2

CARROT LAMB ROAST

Preparation Time: 10 minutes
Cooking Time: 40 minutes
Servings: 4
Ingredients:

- 1-pound lamb loin
- 1 carrot, chopped
- 1 teaspoon dried thyme

- 2 tablespoons coconut oil
- 1 teaspoon salt

Directions:

1. Put all ingredients in the baking tray, mix well.
2. Bake the mixture in the preheated to 360F oven for 40 minutes.

Nutrition:
Calories 295
Fat 17.9
Fiber 0.5
Carbs 1.7
Protein 30.3

LAMB AND CELERY CASSEROLE

Preparation Time: 10 minutes
Cooking Time: 45 minutes
Servings: 2
Ingredients:

- ¼ cup celery stalk, chopped
- 2 lamb chops, chopped
- ½ cup Mozzarella, shredded
- 1 teaspoon butter
- ¼ cup coconut cream
- 1 teaspoon taco seasonings

Directions:

1. Mix lamb chops with taco seasonings and put in the casserole mold.
2. Add celery stalk, coconut cream, and shredded mozzarella.
3. Then add butter and cook the casserole in the preheated to 360F oven for 45 minutes.

Nutrition:
Calories 283
Fat 19.3
Fiber 0.9
Carbs 3.3
Protein 24.8

LAMB IN ALMOND SAUCE

Preparation Time: 10 minutes
Cooking Time: 30 minutes
Servings: 6
Ingredients:

- 14 oz. lamb fillet, cubed
- 1 cup organic almond milk
- 1 teaspoon almond flour
- 1 teaspoon ground nutmeg
- ½ teaspoon ground cardamom
- 1 tablespoon olive oil
- 1 tablespoon lemon juice
- 1 tablespoon butter
- ½ teaspoon minced garlic

Directions:

1. Preheat the olive oil in the saucepan.
2. Meanwhile, mix lamb, ground nutmeg, ground cardamom, and minced garlic.
3. Put the lamb in the hot olive oil. Roast the meat for 2 minutes per side.
4. Then add butter, lemon juice, and almond milk. Carefully mix the mixture.
5. Cook the meal for 15 minutes on medium heat.

6.   Then add almond flour, stir well and simmer the meal for 10 minutes more.

Nutrition:
Calories 258
Fat 19
Fiber 1.1
Carbs 2.7
Protein 19.7

SWEET LEG OF LAMB

Preparation Time: 10 minutes
Cooking Time: 45 minutes
Servings: 6
Ingredients:

- 2 pounds lamb leg
- 1 tablespoon Erythritol
- 3 tablespoons coconut milk
- 1 teaspoon chili flakes
- 1 teaspoon ground turmeric
- 1 teaspoon cayenne pepper
- 3 tablespoons coconut oil

Directions:

1.   In the shallow bowl, mix cayenne pepper, ground turmeric, chili flakes, and Erythritol.
2.   Rub the lamb leg with spices.
3.   Melt the coconut oil in the saucepan.
4.   Add lamb leg and roast it for 10 minutes per side on low heat.
5.   After this, add coconut milk and cook the meal for 30 minutes on low heat. Flip the meat on another side from time to time.

Nutrition:
Calories 350
Fat 18.8
Fiber 0.3
Carbs 0.8
Protein 42.8

COCONUT LAMB SHOULDER

Preparation Time: 10 minutes
Cooking Time: 75 minutes
Servings: 5
Ingredients:

- 2-pound lamb shoulder
- 1 teaspoon ground cumin
- 2 tablespoons butter
- ¼ cup of coconut milk
- 1 teaspoon coconut shred
- ½ cup kale, chopped

Directions:

1.   Put all ingredients in the saucepan and mix well.
2.   Close the lid and cook the meal on low heat for 75 minutes.

Nutrition:
Calories 414
Fat 21.2
Fiber 0.5
Carbs 1.7
Protein 51.5

LAVENDER LAMB

Preparation Time: 10 minutes
Cooking Time: 35 minutes
Servings: 4
Ingredients:

- 4 lamb chops
- 1 teaspoon dried lavender
- 2 tablespoons butter
- 1 teaspoon cumin seeds
- 1 cup of water

Directions:

1.   Toss the butter in the saucepan and melt it.
2.   Add lamb chops and roast them for 3 minutes.
3.   Then add dried lavender, cumin seeds, and water.
4.   Close the lid and cook the meat for 30 minutes on medium-low heat.

Nutrition:
Calories 211 Fat 12.1
Fiber 0.1 Carbs 0.2 Protein 24

DILL LAMB SHANK

Preparation Time: 10 minutes
Cooking Time: 40 minutes
Servings: 3
Ingredients:

- 3 lamb shanks (4 oz. each)
- 1 tablespoon dried dill
- 1 teaspoon peppercorns
- 3 cups of water
- 1 carrot, chopped
- 1 teaspoon salt

Directions:

1.   Bring the water to boil.
2.   Add lamb shank, dried dill, peppercorns, carrot, and salt.
3.   Close the lid and cook the meat in medium heat for 40 minutes.

Nutrition:
Calories 224 Fat 84
Fiber 0.8 Carbs 3 Protein 32.3

MEXICAN LAMB CHOPS

Preparation Time: 10 minutes
Cooking Time: 15 minutes
Servings: 4
Ingredients:

- 4 lamb chops
- 1 tablespoon Mexican seasonings
- 2 tablespoons sesame oil
- 1 teaspoon butter

Directions:

1.   Rub the lamb chops with Mexican seasonings.
2.   Then melt the butter in the skillet. Add sesame oil.
3.   Then add lamb chops and roast them for 7 minutes per side on medium heat.

Nutrition:
Calories 323 Fat 14
Fiber 0 Carbs 1.1 Protein 24.1

CHAPTER 19:

SEAFOOD

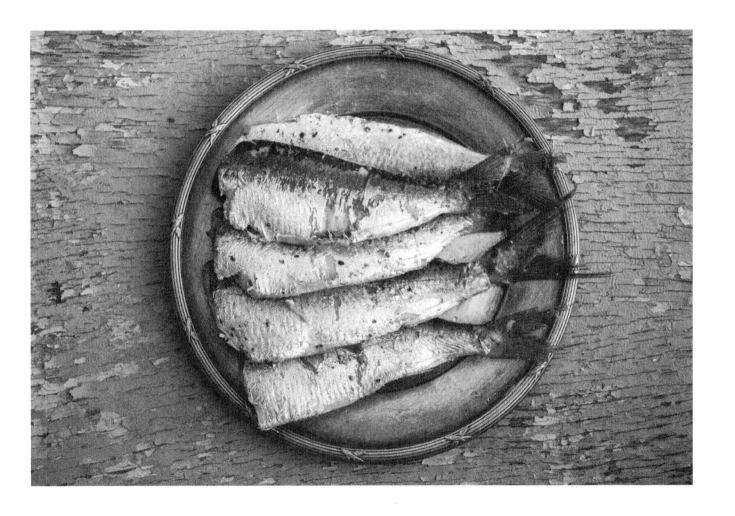

KETO SNACK BARS
INGREDIENTS

- 85g (1/2 cup) almonds
- 55g (1/2 cup) walnut halves
- 80g (1/2 cup) macadamia nuts
- 80g (1/2 cup) pepitas
- 85g (1 cup) desiccated coconut
- One teaspoon ground cinnamon
- 130g (1/2 cup) peanut coconut spread
- 60g (1/4 cup) solidified coconut oil
- Two teaspoons vanilla bean paste

METHOD

Light grate and line with baking paper a 16 x 26 cm (base measurement) lamington saucepan.

In a food processor, process almonds, walnuts, macadamia nuts and pepitas until badly sliced.

Take it into a large tub. Mix the cocoon and cinnamon together.

In a small saucepan add the peanuts, cocoon oil and vanilla and cook, stirring, for 3-5 minutes over low heat or until melted, well combined.

Attach the peanut mix to the dry ingredients and blend well. Press the mixture tightly into the ready pan with the back of a spoon smoothing surface.

Cover and put for 2-3 hours or until firm in the refrigerator. Split into 16 bars. Split into 16 bars.

KETO FISH AND CHIPS
INGREDIENTS

- Two eggs
- One tablespoon pouring cream
- 155g (1 1/2 cups) almond meal
- 40g (1/2 cup) finely grated parmesan cheese
- One large lemon, rind finely grated
- 1/3 cup chopped fresh continental parsley
- One teaspoon dried chilli flakes (optional)
- Two avocados
- Two large zucchini, cut into long wedges
- 4 x 125g skinless firm white fish fillets
- 80ml (1/3 cup) rice bran oil
- Mixed salad leaves, to serve
- Lemon wedges, to serve

METHOD

Preheat oven forced to 220C/200C fan. Cover a large bakery with bakery paper.

In a wide shallow cup, whisk the eggs, cream and one tbs of water. In a shallow bowl, combine almond meal, cheese, rind, parsley and chilli flakes. Saison. Saison.

Cut each avocado half, remove the stone, peel the skin away and cut it into 6-8 wedges.

Working with 1 part at a time, cover a piece of avocado in the mixture of eggs so that excess can spill off and cover into the mixture of almonds. Repeat with the courgettes and shrimp. Spread the crumbed avocado and courgette over a prepared tray evenly. On a plate, cover the crumbed fish and place it in the refrigerator for 10 minutes to rest.

Spray generously with oil the crumbed avocado and zucchini. Bake until golden and crisp for 20 minutes or until black.

Heat the oil over medium-high heat in a large non-stick frying dish. Cook fish on both sides for 2-3 minutes or until golden and crisp. Serve with salad leaves and lemon wedges, fish and chips.

KETO CHICKEN COCONUT CURRY WITH BROCCOLI RICE
INGREDIENTS

- Two tablespoons macadamia oil
- 600g Lilydale Free Range Chicken Thigh, cut into 3cm pieces
- One brown onion, sliced
- Two garlic cloves, crushed
- Two teaspoons finely grated fresh ginger
- Two long red chillies, finely chopped, plus extra sliced to serve
- 1/2 teaspoon turmeric
- Two teaspoons brown mustard seeds
- Two teaspoons ground cumin
- One teaspoon ground coriander
- 400ml can coconut cream
- 500g broccoli, chopped
- Lime juice, to taste
- Fish sauce, to taste
- 100g baby spinach leaves

METHOD

In a big saucepan, heat half the oil, or wok over high heat. Attach half the chicken and cook, sometimes stirring, or browning, for 2-3 minutes. Move to board. Switch to board. Undo the rest of the food.

Add the rest of the oil and the onion to the pot. Cook, stirring, or until soft for 3-4 minutes. Stir in garlic, chilli, ginger, turmeric, mustard, cumin and coriander. Cook, stirring, or until aromatic, for 2 minutes. Add the chicken and the coconut milk. Bring to boil. Bring to boil. Cover partly and rising heat to low. Simmer until chicken is tender for 20 minutes.

In the meantime, process the broccoli, if necessary, in batches, in the food processor until finely chopped and close to rice. Move the broccoli to a large secure microwave dish. Cover and microwave 2-3 minutes or tender on HIGH.

Take heat and season curry with lime juice and fish sauce, to taste. Sprinkle with the spinach and additional chilli and eat rice broccoli.

KETO STRAWBERRY, ALMOND AND CHOCOLATE MUFFINS
INGREDIENTS

- 25g (1/4 cup) coconut flour
- Three teaspoons baking powder

- 200g (2 cups) almond meal
- 50g (1/4 cup) powdered stevia sweetener
- 250g strawberries, hulled, chopped
- 75g dark chocolate (85% cocoa), chopped
- Three eggs, lightly whisked
- Two teaspoons vanilla extract
- 60ml (1/4 cup) almond milk
- 125g unsalted butter, melted

METHOD

Preheat oven forced to 170C/150C fan. Line 12 holes with a capacity of 80ml (1/3 cup) muffin pan with the paper case.

Take a big bowl with the coconut flour and the baking powder.

Remove the meal of the nuts, stevia, strawberries and chocolate and blend together.

Whisk in a tub the bacon, coffee and almond milk.

Add the egg and butter to the dry ingredients and blend until combined.

Divide the mixture between the prepared muffin pants.

Bake in the middle for 20-25 minutes or until the skewer is gold and clean.

Lift for 5 minutes, cool, and cool before moving to a wire rack.

FISH AND EGG PLATE

Preparation Time: 5 minutes;
Cooking Time: 10 minutes;
Servings: 2
Ingredients

- 2 eggs
- 1 tbsp. butter, unsalted
- 2 pacific whitening fillets
- ½ oz. chopped lettuce
- 1 scallion, chopped
- Seasoning:
- 3 tbsp. avocado oil
- 1/3 tsp salt
- 1/3 tsp ground black pepper

Directions:

1. Cook the eggs and for this, take a frying pan, place it over medium heat, add butter and when it melts, crack the egg in the pan and cook for 2 to 3 minutes until fried to desired liking.
2. Transfer fried egg to a plate and then cook the remaining egg in the same manner.
3. Meanwhile, season fish fillets with ¼ tsp each of salt and black pepper.
4. When eggs have fried, sprinkle salt and black pepper on them, then add 1 tbsp. oil into the frying pan, add fillets and cook for 4 minutes per side until thoroughly cooked.
5. When done, distribute fillets to the plate, add lettuce and scallion, drizzle with remaining oil, and then serve.

SESAME TUNA SALAD

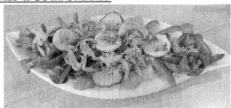

Preparation Time: 35 minutes
Cooking Time: 0 minutes;
Servings: 2
Ingredients

- 6 oz. of tuna in water
- ½ tbsp. chili-garlic paste
- ½ tbsp. black sesame seeds, toasted
- 2 tbsp. mayonnaise
- 1 tbsp. sesame oil
- Seasoning:
- 1/8 tsp red pepper flakes

Directions:

1. Take a medium bowl, all the ingredients for the salad in it except for tuna, and then stir until well combined.
2. Fold in tuna until mixed and then refrigerator for 30 minutes.
3. Serve.

Nutrition: 322 Calories; 25.4 g Fats; 17.7 g Protein; 2.6 g Net Carb; 3 g Fiber;

KETO TUNA SANDWICH

Preparation Time: 10 minutes
Cooking Time: 10 minutes;
Servings: 2
Ingredients

- 2 oz. tuna, packed in water
- 2 2/3 tbsp. coconut flour
- 1 tsp baking powder
- 2 eggs
- 2 tbsp. mayonnaise
- Seasoning:
- 1/4 tsp salt
- 1/4 tsp ground black pepper

Directions:

1. Turn on the oven, then set it to 375 degrees F and let it preheat.
2. Meanwhile, prepare the batter for this, add all the ingredients in a bowl, reserving mayonnaise, 1 egg, and 1/8 tsp salt, and then whisk until well combined.
3. Take a 4 by 4 inches heatproof baking pan, grease it with oil, pour in the prepared batter and bake 10 minutes until bread is firm.
4. Meanwhile, prepare tuna and for this, place tuna in a medium bowl, add mayonnaise, season with remaining salt and black pepper, and then stir until combined.
5. When done, let the bread cool in the pan for 5 minutes, then transfer it to a wire rack and cool for 20 minutes.
6. Slice the bread, prepare sandwiches with prepared tuna mixture, and then serve.

Nutrition: 255 Calories; 17.8 g Fats; 16.3 g Protein; 3.7 g Net Carb; 3.3 g Fiber;

TUNA MELT JALAPENO PEPPERS

Preparation Time: 5 minutes
Cooking Time: 10 minutes;
Servings: 2
Ingredients

- 4 jalapeno peppers
- 1-ounce tuna, packed in water
- 1-ounce cream cheese softened
- 1 tbsp. grated parmesan cheese
- 1 tbsp. grated mozzarella cheese
- Seasoning:
- 1 tsp chopped dill pickles
- 1 green onion, green part sliced only

Directions:

1. Turn on the oven, then set it to 400 degrees F and let it preheat.
2. Prepare the peppers and for this, cut each pepper in half lengthwise and remove seeds and stem.
3. Take a small bowl, place tuna in it, add remaining ingredients except for cheeses, and then stir until combined.
4. Spoon tuna mixture into peppers, sprinkle cheeses on top, and then bake for 7 to 10 minutes until cheese has turned golden brown.
5. Serve.

Nutrition: 104 Calories; 6.2 g Fats; 7 g Protein; 2.1 g Net Carb; 1.1 g Fiber;

SMOKED SALMON FAT BOMBS

Preparation Time: 5 minutes
Cooking Time: 0 minutes;
Servings: 2
Ingredients

- 2 tbsp. cream cheese, softened
- 1 ounce smoked salmon
- 2 tsp bagel seasoning

Directions:

1. Take a medium bowl, place cream cheese and salmon in it, and stir until well combined.
2. Shape the mixture into bowls, roll them into bagel seasoning and then serve.

Nutrition: 65 Calories; 4.8 g Fats; 4 g Protein; 0.5 g Net Carb; 0 g Fiber;

SALMON CUCUMBER ROLLS

Preparation Time: 15 minutes;
Cooking Time: 0 minutes;
Servings: 2
Ingredients

- 1 large cucumber
- 2 oz. smoked salmon
- 4 tbsp. mayonnaise
- 1 tsp sesame seeds
- Seasoning:
- ¼ tsp salt
- ¼ tsp ground black pepper

Directions:

1. Trim the ends of the cucumber, cut it into slices by using a vegetable peeler, and then place half of the cucumber slices in a dish.
2. Cover with paper towels, layer with remaining cucumber slices, top with paper towels, and let them refrigerate for 5 minutes.
3. Meanwhile, take a medium bowl, place salmon in it, add mayonnaise, season with salt and black pepper, and then stir until well combined.
4. Remove cucumber slices from the refrigerator, place salmon on one side of each cucumber slice, and then roll tightly.
5. Repeat with remaining cucumber, sprinkle with sesame seeds and then serve.

Nutrition: 269 Calories; 24 g Fats; 6.7 g Protein; 4 g Net Carb; 2 g Fiber;

BACON WRAPPED MAHI-MAHI

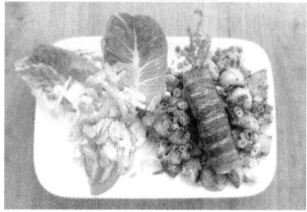

Preparation Time: 10 minutes
Cooking Time: 12 minutes;
Servings: 2
Ingredients

- 2 fillets of mahi-mahi
- 2 strips of bacon - ½ of lime, zested
- 4 basil leaves - ½ tsp salt
- Seasoning:
- ½ tsp ground black pepper
- 1 tbsp. avocado oil

Directions:

1. Turn on the oven, then set it to 375 degrees F and let them preheat. Meanwhile, season fillets with salt and black pepper, top each fillet with 2 basil leaves, sprinkle with lime zest, wrap with a bacon strip and secure with a toothpick if needed. Take a medium skillet pan, place it over medium-high heat, add oil and when hot, place prepared fillets in it and cook for 2 minutes per side.
2. Transfer pan into the oven and bake the fish for 5 to 7 minutes until thoroughly cooked.
3. Serve.

Nutrition: 217 Calories; 11.3 g Fats; 27.1 g Protein; 1.2 g Net Carb; 0.5 g Fiber;

CHEESY GARLIC BREAD WITH SMOKED SALMON

Preparation Time: 10 minutes
Cooking Time: 1 minute;
Servings: 2
Ingredients

- 4 tbsp. almond flour
- ½ tsp baking powder

- 2 tbsp. grated cheddar cheese
- 1 egg
- 2 oz. salmon, cut into thin sliced
- Seasoning:
- 1 tbsp. butter, unsalted
- ¼ tsp garlic powder
- 1/8 tsp salt
- ¼ tsp Italian seasoning

Directions:

1. Take a heatproof bowl, place all the ingredients in it except for cheese and then stir by using a fork until well combined.
2. Fold in cheese until just mixed and then microwave for 1 minute at high heat setting until thoroughly cooked, else continue cooking for another 15 to 30 seconds.
3. When done, lift out the bread, cool it for 5 minutes and then cut it into slices.
4. Top each slice with salmon and then serve straight away

Nutrition: 233 Calories; 18 g Fats; 13.8 g Protein; 1.9 g Net Carb; 1.5 g Fiber;

SMOKED SALMON PASTA SALAD

Preparation Time: 10 minutes
Cooking Time: 0 minutes;
Servings: 2
Ingredients

- 1 zucchini, spiralized into noodles
- 4 oz. smoked salmon, break into pieces
- 2 oz. cream cheese
- 2 oz. mayonnaise
- 2 oz. sour cream
- Seasoning:
- 1/3 tsp salt
- ¼ tsp ground black pepper
- ¼ tsp hot sauce

Directions:

1. Take a medium bowl, place cream cheese in it, add mayonnaise, sour cream, salt, black pepper and hot sauce and stir until well combined.
2. Add zucchini noodles, toss until well coated and then fold in salmon until just mixed.
3. Serve.

Nutrition: 458 Calories; 38.7 g Fats; 15.4 g Protein; 6.1 g Net Carb; 1.7 g Fiber;

TUNA SALAD PICKLE BOATS

Preparation Time: 10 minutes
Cooking Time: 0 minutes;
Servings: 2
Ingredients

- 4 dill pickles
- 4 oz. of tuna, packed in water, drained
- ¼ of lime, juiced
- 4 tbsp. mayonnaise
- Seasoning:
- ¼ tsp salt
- 1/8 tsp ground black pepper
- ¼ tsp paprika
- 1 tbsp. mustard paste

Directions:

1. Prepare tuna salad and for this, take a medium bowl, place tuna in it, add lime juice, mayonnaise, salt, black pepper, paprika, and mustard and stir until mixed.
2. Cut each pickle into half lengthwise, scoop out seeds, and then fill with tuna salad.
3. Serve.

Nutrition: 308.5 Calories; 23.7 g Fats; 17 g Protein; 3.8 g Net Carb; 3.1 g Fiber;

SHRIMP DEVILED EGGS

Preparation Time: 5 minutes
Cooking Time: 0 minutes;
Servings: 2
Ingredients

- 2 eggs, boiled
- 2 oz. shrimps, cooked, chopped
- ½ tsp tabasco sauce
- ½ tsp mustard paste
- 2 tbsp. mayonnaise
- Seasoning:
- 1/8 tsp salt
- 1/8 tsp ground black pepper

Directions:

1. Peel the boiled eggs, then slice in half lengthwise and transfer egg yolks to a medium bowl by using a spoon.
2. Mash the egg yolk, add remaining ingredients and stir until well combined.
3. Spoon the egg yolk mixture into egg whites, and then serve.

Nutrition: 210 Calories; 16.4 g Fats; 14 g Protein; 1 g Net Carb; 0.1 g Fiber;

HERB CRUSTED TILAPIA

Preparation Time: 5 minutes
Cooking Time: 10 minutes;
Servings: 2
Ingredients

- 2 fillets of tilapia
- ½ tsp garlic powder
- ½ tsp Italian seasoning
- ½ tsp dried parsley
- 1/3 tsp salt
- Seasoning:
- 2 tbsp. melted butter, unsalted
- 1 tbsp. avocado oil

Directions:

1. Turn on the broiler and then let it preheat.
2. Meanwhile, take a small bowl, place melted butter in it, stir in oil and garlic powder until mixed, and then brush this mixture over tilapia fillets.
3. Stir together remaining spices and then sprinkle them generously on tilapia until well coated.
4. Place seasoned tilapia in a baking pan, place the pan under the broiler and then bake for 10 minutes until tender and golden, brushing with garlic-butter every 2 minutes.
5. Serve.

Nutrition: 520 Calories; 35 g Fats; 36.2 g Protein; 13.6 g Net Carb; 0.6 g Fiber;

TUNA STUFFED AVOCADO

Preparation Time: 5 minutes
Cooking Time: 0 minutes;
Servings: 2
Ingredients

- 1 medium avocado
- ¼ of a lemon, juiced
- 5-ounce tuna, packed in water
- 1 green onion, chopped
- 2 slices of turkey bacon, cooked, crumbled
- Seasoning:
- ¼ tsp salt
- ¼ tsp ground black pepper

Directions:

1. Drain tuna, place it in a bowl, and then broke it into pieces with a form.
2. Add remaining ingredients, except for avocado and bacon, and stir until well combined.
3. Cut avocado into half, remove its pit and then stuff its cavity evenly with the tuna mixture.
4. Top stuffed avocados with bacon and Serve.

Nutrition: 108.5 Calories; 8 g Fats; 6 g Protein; 0.8 g Net Carb; 2.3 g Fiber;

GARLIC BUTTER SALMON

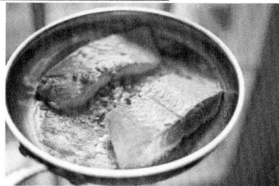

Preparation Time: 10 minutes
Cooking Time: 15 minutes
Servings: 2
Ingredients

- 2 salmon fillets, skinless
- 1 tsp minced garlic
- 1 tbsp. chopped cilantro
- 1 tbsp. unsalted butter
- 2 tbsp. grated cheddar cheese
- Seasoning:
- ½ tsp salt
- ¼ tsp ground black pepper

Directions:

1. Turn on the oven, then set it to 350 degrees F, and let it preheat.
2. Meanwhile, taking a rimmed baking sheet, grease it with oil, place salmon fillets on it, season with salt and black pepper on both sides.
3. Stir together butter, cilantro, and cheese until combined, then coat the mixture on both sides of salmon in an even layer and bake for 15 minutes until thoroughly cooked.
4. Then Turn on the broiler and continue baking the salmon for 2 minutes until the top is golden brown.
5. Serve.

Nutrition: 128 Calories; 4.5 g Fats; 41 g Protein; 1 g Net Carb; 0 g Fiber;

CHAPTER 20:

VEGETABLES

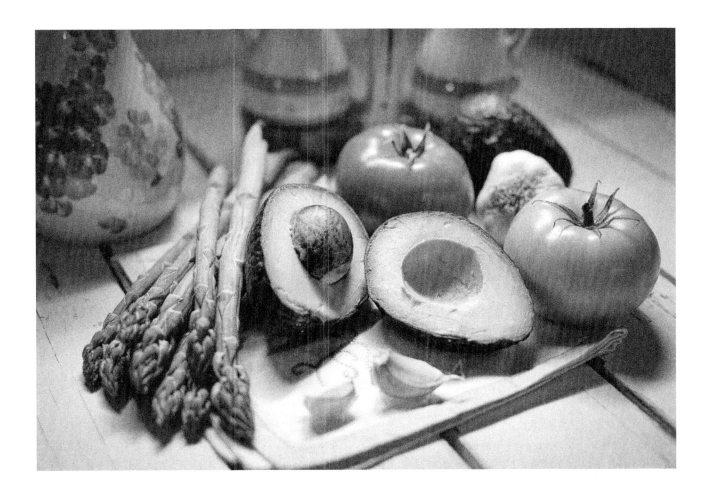

KOTO DIET RECIPES

Keto taco shells

INGREDIENTS

- 60g (2 cups, firmly packed) baby spinach leaves
- Two eggs
- 40g (1/3 cup) almond meal
- Two teaspoons psyllium husk
- 1/2 teaspoon salt

METHOD

Preheat oven forced to 180C/160C fan. Bakery Line 2 with bakery paper.

Place the spinach in a heat-resistant bath. Pour over hot water to cover. To cover. Set aside to blanch for 5 minutes. Drain, squeeze out extra oil.

Move the spinach to a food processor's tank. Remove the seeds, almond milk, husk and salt. Method to smoothness. Place one-quarter of the mixture on one of the trays prepared. Using a spatula to spread to form a circle of 15 cm. Repeat 4 circles with the remaining mixture.

Bake until set for 10 minutes.

To build a taco shape, use a spatula to move the cycles between the gaps in an upturning non-stick muffin pot.

Set aside for a little cooling. Bake to dry for another 10 minutes.

Load your favourite ingredients with a taco.

ONE-POT KETO ZUCCHINI ALFRED

INGREDIENTS

- One tablespoon extra-virgin olive oil
- 15g butter
- 2 x 250g packets zucchini noodles
- Two garlic cloves, finely chopped
- 100g cream cheese, chopped
- One tablespoon thickened cream
- 20g (1/4 cup) finely grated parmesan, (or vegetarian hard cheese) plus extra to serve

METHOD

In a frying pan, heat the oil and butter over medium heat until the butter is foamy. Add the noodles of zucchini. Use tongs for 1-2 minutes occasionally or slightly wilted. Using moving tongs to a pot.

Fill the pan with the garlic. Cook, stirring, or until aromatic for 1 minute. Stir in milk, cream and 60ml (1/4 cup) of tea. Reduce to the low sun. Cook, often stirring, for 3 minutes or until smooth. Remove the parmesan and the season. Attach the zucchini and mix with tongs. Serve with extra parmesan.

LOADED CAULIFLOWER MASH

INGREDIENTS

- One large cauliflower, trimmed, cut in florets
- Two garlic cloves, peeled, smashed
- One tablespoon olive oil
- 200g streaky bacon, coarsely chopped
- 85g (1/3 cup) sour cream

- 80g (1 cup) coarsely grated cheddar
- One tablespoon chopped fresh chives, plus extra to sprinkle
- Melted butter, to serve

METHOD

Bring to the boil a large bowl of water. Attach the chocolate and garlic and cook for 10-15 minutes or until the chocolate is warm. Drain and dry with a towel or cloth. Alternatively, heat the oil over medium heat in the frying pan. Add bacon and cook until golden and crisp for four minutes. Set aside. Set aside.

Preheat oven to fan-forced 180C/160C. In a food processor, process the cauliflower mixture until it forms thin crumbs. Take a medium bowl. Cut the savoury sauce, part of the cheese and chives.

In around 20 cm ovenproof dish, place the cauliflower mixture. Finish the remainder of the cheese with the bacon. Bake until cheese is melted and crispy for 10 minutes or without cooking. Sprinkle with additional sprinkles. Drizzle with butter. Butter. In the meantime, heat the oil over medium heat in the frying pan. Remove bacon and cook for 4 minutes, or until crisp and golden. Set aside. Set aside.

Preheat oven to fan-forced 180C/160C. In a food processor, process the cauliflower mixture until it forms thin crumbs. Take a medium bowl. Cut the savoury sauce, part of the cheese and chives.

In around 20 cm ovenproof dish, place the cauliflower mixture. Finish the remainder of the cheese with the bacon. Bake until cheese is melted and crispy for 10 minutes or without cooking. Sprinkle with additional sprinkles. Drizzle with butter. Butter.

PORTOBELLO MUSHROOM PIZZA

Preparation Time: 15 minutes
Cooking Time: 5 minutes
Servings: 4
Ingredients:

- 4 large portobello mushrooms, stems removed
- ¼ cup olive oil
- 1 teaspoon minced garlic
- 1 medium tomato, cut into 4 slices
- 2 teaspoons chopped fresh basil
- 1 cup shredded mozzarella cheese

Directions:

1. Preheat the oven to broil. Line a baking sheet with aluminum foil and set aside.
2. In a small bowl, toss the mushroom caps with the olive oil until well coated. Use your fingertips to rub the oil in without breaking the mushrooms.
3. Place the mushrooms on the baking sheet gill-side down and broil the mushrooms until they are tender on the tops, about 2 minute
4. Flip the mushrooms over and broil 1 minute more
5. Take the baking sheet out and spread the garlic over each mushroom, top each with a tomato slice, sprinkle with the basil, and top with the cheese

6. Broil the mushrooms until the cheese is melted and bubbly, about 1 minute.
7. Serve.

Nutrition:
Calories: 251
Fat: 20g
Protein: 14g
Carbs: 7g
Fiber: 3g Net Carbs: 4g
Fat 71 Protein 19
Carbs 10

GARLICKY GREEN BEANS

Preparation Time: 10 minutes
Cooking Time: 10 minutes
Servings: 4
Ingredients:

- 1 pound green beans, stemmed
- 2 tablespoons olive oil
- 1 teaspoon minced garlic
- Sea salt
- Freshly ground black pepper
- ¼ cup freshly grated Parmesan cheese

Directions:

1. Preheat the oven to 425°F. Line a baking sheet with aluminum foil and set aside.
2. In a large bowl, toss together the green beans, olive oil, and garlic until well mixed.
3. Season the beans lightly with salt and pepper
4. Spread the beans on the baking sheet and roast them until they are tender and lightly browned, stirring them once, about 10 minutes.
5. Serve topped with the Parmesan cheese.

Nutrition:
Calories: 104 Fat: 9g
Protein: 4g Carbs: 2g
Fiber: 1g Net Carbs: 1g
Fat 77 Protein 15
Carbs 8

SAUTÉED ASPARAGUS WITH WALNUTS

Preparation Time: 10 minutes
Cooking Time: 5 minutes
Servings: 4
Ingredients:

- 1½ tablespoons olive oil
- ¾ pound asparagus, woody ends trimmed
- Sea salt
- Freshly ground pepper
- ¼ cup chopped walnuts

Directions:

1. Place a large skillet over medium-high heat and add the olive oil.
2. Sauté the asparagus until the spears are tender and lightly browned, about 5 minutes.
3. Season the asparagus with salt and pepper.
4. Remove the skillet from the heat and toss the asparagus with the walnuts.
5. Serve.

Nutrition:
Calories: 124 Fat: 12g
Protein: 3g Carbs: 4g
Fiber: 2g
Net Carbs: 2g
Fat 81
Protein
Carbs 10

BRUSSELS SPROUTS CASSEROLE

Preparation Time: 15 minutes
Cooking Time: 30 minutes
Servings: 8
Ingredients:

- 8 bacon slices
- 1 pound Brussels sprouts, blanched for 10 minutes and cut into quarters
- 1 cup shredded Swiss cheese, divided
- ¾ cup heavy (whipping) cream

Directions:

1. Preheat the oven to 400°F.
2. Place a skillet over medium-high heat and cook the bacon until it is crispy, about 6 minutes.
3. Reserve 1 tablespoon of bacon fat to grease the casserole dish and roughly chop the cooked bacon.
4. Lightly oil a casserole dish with the reserved bacon fat and set aside.
5. In a medium bowl, toss the Brussels sprouts with the chopped bacon and ½ cup of cheese and transfer the mixture to the casserole dish.
6. Pour the heavy cream over the Brussels sprouts and top the casserole with the remaining ½ cup of cheese.
7. Bake until the cheese is melted and lightly browned and the vegetables are heated through, about 20 minutes.
8. Serve.

Nutrition:
Calories: 299
Fat: 11g
Protein: 12g
Carbs: 7g
Fiber: 3g
Net Carbs: 4g
Fat 77
Protein 15
Carbs 8

CREAMED SPINACH

Preparation Time: 10 minutes
Cooking Time: 30 minutes
Servings: 4
Ingredients:

- 1 tablespoon butter
- ½ sweet onion, very thinly sliced
- 4 cups spinach, stemmed and thoroughly washed
- ¾ cup heavy (whipping) cream
- ¼ cup Herbed Chicken Stock (here)
- Pinch sea salt
- Pinch freshly ground black pepper
- Pinch ground nutmeg

Directions:

1. In a large skillet over medium heat, add the butter.

2. Sauté the onion until it is lightly caramelized, about 5 minutes.
3. Stir in the spinach, heavy cream, chicken stock, salt, pepper, and nutmeg.
4. Sauté until the spinach is wilted, about 5 minutes.
5. Continue cooking the spinach until it is tender and the sauce is thickened, about 15 minutes.
6. Serve immediately.

Nutrition:
Calories: 195
Fat: 20g
Protein: 3g
Carbs: 3g
Fiber: 2g
Net Carbs: 1g
Fat 88
Protein 6
Carbs 6

CHEESY MASHED CAULIFLOWER

Preparation Time: 15 minutes
Cooking Time: 5 minutes
Servings: 4
Ingredients:
- 1 head cauliflower, chopped roughly
- ½ cup shredded Cheddar cheese
- ¼ cup heavy (whipping) cream
- 2 tablespoons butter, at room temperature
- Sea salt
- Freshly ground black pepper

Directions:
1. Place a large saucepan filled three-quarters full with water over high heat and bring to a boil.
2. Blanch the cauliflower until tender, about 5 minutes, and drain.
3. Transfer the cauliflower to a food processor and add the cheese, heavy cream, and butter. Purée until very creamy and whipped.
4. Season with salt and pepper.
5. Serve.

Nutrition:
Calories: 183
Fat: 15g
Protein: 8g
Carbs: 6g
Fiber: 2g
Net Carbs: 4g
Fat 75
Protein 14
Carbs 11

SAUTÉED CRISPY ZUCCHINI

Preparation Time: 15 minutes
Cooking Time: 10 minutes
Servings: 4
Ingredients:
- 2 tablespoons butter
- 4 zucchini, cut into ¼-inch-thick rounds
- ½ cup freshly grated Parmesan cheese
- Freshly ground black pepper

Directions:
1. Place a large skillet over medium-high heat and melt the butter.
2. Add the zucchini and sauté until tender and lightly browned, about 5 minutes.
3. Spread the zucchini evenly in the skillet and sprinkle the Parmesan cheese over the vegetables.
4. Cook without stirring until the Parmesan cheese is melted and crispy where it touches the skillet, about 5 minutes.
5. Serve.

Nutrition:
Calories: 94
Fat: 8g
Protein: 4g
Carbs: 1g
Fiber: 0g
Net Carbs: 1g
Fat 76
Protein 20
Carbs 4

MUSHROOMS WITH CAMEMBERT

Preparation Time: 5 minutes
Cooking Time: 15 minutes
Servings: 4
Ingredients:
- 2 tablespoons butter
- 2 teaspoons minced garlic
- 1 pound button mushrooms, halved
- 4 ounces Camembert cheese, diced
- Freshly ground black pepper

Directions:
1. Place a large skillet over medium-high heat and melt the butter.
2. Sauté the garlic until translucent, about 3 minutes.
3. Sauté the mushrooms until tender, about 10 minutes.
4. Stir in the cheese and sauté until melted, about 2 minutes.
5. Season with pepper and serve.

Nutrition:
Calories: 161
Fat: 13g
Protein: 9g
Carbs: 4g
Fiber: 1g
Net Carbs: 3g
Fat 70
Protein 21
Carbs 9

PESTO ZUCCHINI NOODLES

Preparation Time: 15 minutes
Cooking Time: 10 minutes
Servings: 4
Ingredients:
- 4 small zucchini, ends trimmed
- ¾ cup Herb Kale Pesto (here)¼ cup grated or shredded
- Parmesan chees

Directions:
1. Use a spiralizer or peeler to cut the zucchini into "noodles" and place them in a medium bowl.

2. Add the pesto and the Parmesan cheese and toss to coat.
3. Serve.

Nutrition:
Calories: 93
Fat: 8g
Protein: 4g
Carbs: 2g
Fiber: 0g
Net Carbs: 2g
Fat 70
Protein 15
Carbs 8

GOLDEN ROSTI

Preparation Time: 15 minutes
Cooking Time: 15 minutes
Servings: 8
Ingredients:

- 8 bacon slices, chopped
- 1 cup shredded acorn squash
- 1 cup shredded raw celeriac
- 2 tablespoons grated or shredded Parmesan cheese
- 2 teaspoons minced garlic
- 1 teaspoon chopped fresh thyme
- Sea salt
- Freshly ground black pepper
- 2 tablespoons butter

Directions:

1. In a large skillet over medium-high heat, cook the bacon until crispy, about 5 minutes.
2. While the bacon is cooking, in a large bowl, mix together the squash, celeriac, Parmesan cheese, garlic, and thyme. Season the mixture generously with salt and pepper, and set aside.
3. Remove the cooked bacon with a slotted spoon to the rosti mixture and stir to incorporate.
4. Remove all but 2 tablespoons of bacon fat from the skillet and add the butter
5. Reduce the heat to medium-low and transfer the rosti mixture to the skillet and spread it out evenly to form a large round patty about 1 inch thick.
6. Cook until the bottom of the rosti is golden brown and crisp, about 5 minutes.
7. Flip the rosti over and cook until the other side is crispy and the middle is cooked through, about 5 minutes more.
8. Remove the skillet from the heat and cut the rosti into 8 pieces
9. Serve.

Nutrition:
Calories: 171
Fat: 15g
Protein: 5g
Carbs: 3g
Fiber: 0g
Net Carbs: 3g
Fat 81
Protein 12
Carbs 7

ARTICHOKE AND AVOCADO PASTA SALAD

Preparation Time: 15 minutes
Cooking Time: 30 minutes
Servings: 10 servings
Ingredients:

- Two cups of spiral pasta (uncooked)
- A quarter cup of Romano cheese (grated)
- One can (fourteen oz.) of artichoke hearts (coarsely chopped and drained well)
- One avocado (medium-sized, ripe, cubed)
- Two plum tomatoes (chopped coarsely)

For the dressing:

- One tbsp. of fresh cilantro (chopped)
- Two tbsps. of lime juice
- A quarter cup of canola oil
- One and a half tsps. of lime zest (grated)
- Half a tsp. each of
- Pepper (freshly ground)
- Kosher salt

Directions:

1. Follow the directions mentioned on the package for cooking the pasta. Drain them well and rinse using cold water.
2. Then, take a large-sized bowl and in it, add the pasta along with the tomatoes, artichoke hearts, cheese, and avocado. Combine them well. Then, take another bowl and add all the ingredients of the dressing in it. Whisk them together and, once combined, add the dressing over the pasta.
3. Gently toss the mixture to coat everything evenly in the dressing and then refrigerate.

Nutrition:
Calories: 188
Protein: 6g
Fat: 10g
Carbs: 21g
Fiber: 2g

APPLE ARUGULA AND TURKEY SALAD IN A JAR

Preparation Time: 10 minutes
Cooking Time: 10 minutes
Servings: 4 servings
Ingredients:

- Three tbsps. of red wine vinegar
- Two tbsps. of chives (freshly minced)
- Half a cup of orange juice
- One to three tbsps. of sesame oil
- A quarter tsp. each of
- Pepper (coarsely ground)
- Salt

For the salad:

- Four tsps. of curry powder
- Four cups each of
- Turkey (cubed, cooked)
- Baby spinach or fresh arugula
- A quarter tsp. of salt
- Half a tsp. of pepper (coarsely ground)
- One cup of halved green grapes
- One apple (large-sized, chopped)

- Eleven oz. of mandarin oranges (properly drained)
- One tbsp. of lemon juice
- Half a cup each of
- Walnuts (chopped)
- Dried cranberries or pomegranate seeds

Directions:

1. Take a small-sized bowl and, in it, add the first 6 ingredients from the list into it. Whisk them. Then take a large bowl and in it, add the turkey and then add the seasonings on top of it. Toss the turkey cubes to coat them with the seasoning. Take another bowl and in it, add the lemon juice and toss the apple chunks in the juice.

2. Take four jars and divide the layers in the order I mention here - first goes the orange juice mixture, the second layer is that of the turkey, then apple, oranges, grapes, cranberries or pomegranate seeds, walnuts, and spinach or arugula. Cover the jars and then refrigerate them.

Nutrition:
Calories: 471
Protein: 45g
Fat: 19g
Carbs: 33g
Fiber: 5g

CHAPTER 21:

SNACKS

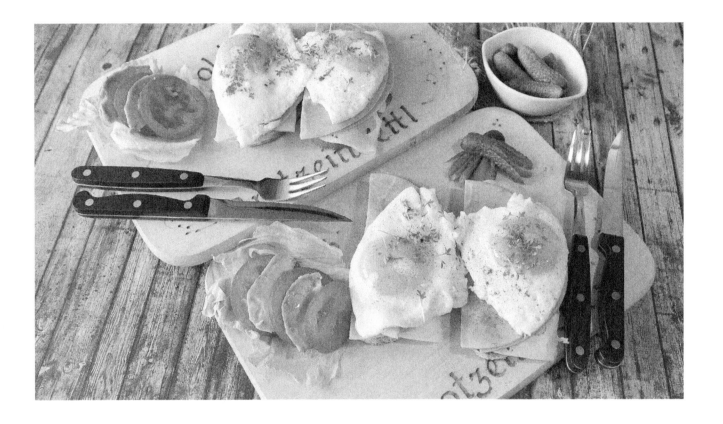

PUMPKIN MUFFINS.

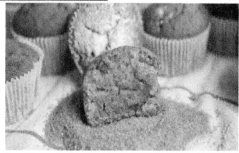

Preparation Time: 10 minutes
Cooking Time: 15 minutes
Servings: 18
Ingredients:
- ¼ cup sunflower seed butter
- ¾ cup pumpkin puree 2 tablespoons flaxseed meal ¼ cup coconut flour
- ½ cup erythritol ½ teaspoon nutmeg, ground
- 1 teaspoon cinnamon, ground ½ teaspoon baking soda 1 egg ½ teaspoon baking powder
- A pinch of salt

Directions:
1. In a bowl, mix butter with pumpkin puree and egg and blend well.
2. Add flaxseed meal, coconut flour, erythritol, baking soda, baking powder, nutmeg, cinnamon and a pinch of salt and stir well.
3. Spoon this into a greased muffin pan, introduce in the oven at 350 degrees F and bake for 15 minutes.
4. Leave muffins to cool down and serve them as a snack.
5. Enjoy!

Nutrition:
Calories: 65 kcal Protein: 2.82 g
Fat: 5.42 g Carbohydrates: 2.27 g
Sodium: 57 mg

CREAMY MANGO AND MINT DIP

Preparation Time: 10 minutes
Cooking Time: 15 minutes
Servings 4
Ingredients:
- Medium green chili, chopped – 1
- Medium white onion, peeled and chopped – 1
- Grated ginger – 1 tablespoon
- Minced garlic – 1 teaspoon
- Salt – 1/8 teaspoon
- Ground black pepper – 1/8 teaspoon
- Cumin powder – 1 teaspoon
- Mango powder – 1 teaspoon
- Mint leaves – 2 cups
- Coriander leaves – 1 cup
- Cashew yogurt – 4 tablespoons

Directions:
1. Place all the ingredients for the dip in a blender and pulse for 1 to 2 minutes or until smooth.
2. Tip the dip into small cups and serve straightaway.

Nutrition: calories: 100, fat: 2, fiber: 3, carbs: 7, protein: 5

HOT RED CHILI AND GARLIC CHUTNEY

Preparation Time: 25 minutes
Cooking Time: 15 minutes
Servings 1
Ingredients:
- Red chilies, dried – 14
- Minced garlic – 5 teaspoons
- Salt – 1/8 teaspoon
- Water – 1 and ¼ cups

Directions:
1. Place chilies in a bowl, pour in water and let rest for 20 minutes.
2. Then drain red chilies, chop them and add to a blender. Add remaining ingredients into the blender and pulse for 1 to 2 minutes until smooth. Tip the sauce into a bowl and serve straight away.

Nutrition: calories: 100, fat: 1, fiber: 2, carbs: 6, protein: 7

RED CHILIES AND ONION CHUTNEY

Preparation Time: 15 minutes
Cooking Time: 15 minutes
Servings 2
Ingredients:
- Medium white onion, peeled and chopped – 1
- Minced garlic – 1 teaspoon
- Red chilies, chopped – 2
- Salt – ¼ teaspoon
- Sweet paprika – 1 teaspoon
- Avocado oil – 2 teaspoons
- Water – ¼ cup

Directions:
1. Place a medium skillet pan over medium-high heat, add oil and when hot, add onion, garlic, and chilies.
2. Cook onions for 5 minutes or until softened, then season with salt and paprika and pour in water. Stir well and cook for 5 minutes. Then spoon the chutney into a bowl and serve.

Nutrition: calories: 121, fat: 2, fiber: 6, carbs: 9, protein: 5

FAST GUACAMOLE

Preparation Time: 10 minutes
Cooking Time: 15 minutes
Servings 12
Ingredients:
- Medium avocados, peeled, pitted and cubed – 3
- Medium tomato, cubed – 1
- Chopped cilantro – ¼ cup
- Medium red onion, peeled and chopped – 1
- Salt – ½ teaspoon
- Ground white pepper – ¼ teaspoon
- Lime juice – 3 tablespoons

Directions:
1. Place all the ingredients for the salad in a medium bowl and stir until combined.
2. Serve guacamole straightaway as an appetizer.

Nutrition: calories: 87, fat: 4, fiber: 4, carbs: 8, protein: 2

COCONUT DILL DIP

Preparation Time: 10 minutes
Cooking Time: 15 minutes
Servings 10
Ingredients:

- Chopped white onion – 1 tablespoon
- Parsley flakes – 2 teaspoons
- Chopped dill – 2 teaspoons
- Salt – ¼ teaspoon
- Coconut cream – 1 cup
- Avocado mayonnaise – ½ cup

Directions:

1. Place all the ingredients for the dip in a medium bowl and whisk until combined.Serve the dip with vegetable sticks as a side dish.

Nutrition: calories: 102, fat: 3, fiber: 1, carbs: 2, protein: 2

CREAMY CRAB DIP

Preparation Time 5 minutes
Cooking Time: 10 minutes
Servings 12
Ingredients:

- Crab meat, chopped – 1 pound
- Chopped white onion – 2 tablespoons
- Minced garlic – 1 tablespoon
- Lemon juice – 2 tablespoons
- Cream cheese, cubed – 16 ounces
- Avocado mayonnaise – 1/3 cup
- Grape juice – 2 tablespoons

Directions:

1. Place all the ingredients for the dip in a medium bowl and stir until combined.
2. Divide dip evenly between small bowls and serve as a party dip.

Nutrition: Calories: 100, Fat: 4, Fiber: 1, Carbs: 4, Protein: 4

CREAMY CHEDDAR AND BACON SPREAD WITH ALMONDS

Preparation Time: 10 minutes
Cooking Time: 10 minutes
Servings 12
Ingredients:

- Bacon, cooked and chopped – 12 ounces
- Chopped sweet red pepper – 2 tablespoons
- Medium white onion, peeled and chopped – 1
- Salt – ¾ teaspoon
- Ground black pepper – ½ teaspoon
- Almonds, chopped – ½ cup
- Cheddar cheese, grated – 1 pound
- Avocado mayonnaise – 2 cups

Directions:

1. Place all the ingredients for the dip in a medium bowl and stir until combined.
2. Divide dip evenly between small bowls and serve as a party dip.

Nutrition: calories: 184, fat: 12, fiber: 1, carbs: 4, protein: 5

GREEN TABASCO DEVILLED EGGS

Preparation Time: 20 minutes
Cooking Time: 10 minutes
Servings: 6
Ingredients:

- 6 Eggs
- 1/3 cup Mayonnaise
- 1 ½ tbsp. Green Tabasco
- Salt and Pepper, to taste

Directions:

1. Place the eggs in a saucepan over medium heat and pour boiling water over, enough to cover them.
2. Cook for 6-8 minutes.
3. Place in an ice bath to cool.
4. When safe to handle, peel the eggs and slice them in half.
5. Scoop out the yolks and place in a bowl.
6. Add the remaining ingredients.
7. Whisk to combine.
8. Fill the egg holes with the mixture.
9. Serve and enjoy!

Nutrition:
Calories 175
Total Fats 17g
Net Carbs: 5g
Protein 6g
Fiber: 1g

HERBED CHEESE BALLS

Preparation Time: 30 MIN
Cooking Time: 10 minutes
Servings: 20
Ingredients:

- 1/3 cup grated Parmesan Cheese
- 3 tbsp. Heavy Cream
- 4 tbsp. Butter, melted
- ¼ tsp Pepper
- 2 Eggs
- 1 cup Almond Flour
- ¼ cup Basil Leaves
- ¼ cup Parsley Leaves
- 2 tbsp. chopped Cilantro Leaves
- 1/3 cup crumbled Feta Cheese

Directions:

1. Place the ingredients in your food processor.
2. Pulse until the mixture becomes smooth.
3. Transfer to a bowl and freeze for 20 minutes or so, to set.
4. Shale the mixture into 20 balls.
5. Meanwhile, preheat the oven to 350 degrees F.
6. Arrange the cheese balls on a lined baking sheet.
7. Place in the oven and bake for 10 minutes.
8. Serve and enjoy!

Nutrition:
Calories 60 Total Fats 5g
Net Carbs: 8g Protein 2g
Fiber: 1g

CHEESY SALAMI SNACK

Preparation Time: 30 MIN
Cooking Time: 10 minutes
Servings: 6
Ingredients:

- 4 ounces Cream Cheese
- 7 ounces dried Salami
- ¼ cup chopped Parsley

Directions:

1. Preheat the oven to 325 degrees F.
2. Slice the salami thinly (I got 30 slices).
3. Arrange the salami on a lined sheet and bake for 15 minutes.
4. Arrange on a serving platter and top each salami slice with a bit of cream cheese.
5. Serve and enjoy!

Nutrition:
Calories 139 Total Fats 15g
Net Carbs: 1g Protein 9g
Fiber: 0g

PESTO & OLIVE FAT BOMBS

Preparation Time: 25 MIN
Cooking Time: 10 minutes
Servings: 8
Ingredients:

- 1 cup Cream Cheese
- 10 Olives, sliced
- 2 tbsp. Pesto Sauce
- ½ cup grated Parmesan Cheese

Directions:

1. Place all of the ingredients in a bowl.
2. Stir well to combine.
3. Place in the freezer and freeze for 15-20 minutes, to set.
4. Shape into 8 balls.
5. Serve and enjoy!

Nutrition:
Calories 123
Total Fats 13g
Net Carbs: 3g
Protein 4g
Fiber: 3g

CHEESY BROCCOLI NUGGETS

Preparation Time: 25 MIN
Cooking Time: 10 minutes
Servings: 4
Ingredients:

- 1 cup shredded Cheese
- ¼ cup Almond Flour
- 2 cups Broccoli Florets, steamed in the microwave for 5 minutes
- 2 Egg Whites
- Salt and Pepper, to taste

Directions:

1. Preheat the oven to 350 degrees F.
2. Place the broccoli florets in a bowl and mash them with a potato masher.
3. Add the remaining ingredients and mix well with your hands, until combined.
4. Line a baking sheet with parchment paper.
5. Drop 20 scoops of the mixture onto the sheet.
6. Place in the oven and bake for 20 minutes or until golden.
7. Serve and enjoy!

Nutrition:
Calories 145
Total Fats 9g
Net Carbs: 4g
Protein 10g
Fiber: 1g

CHAPTER 22:

DESSERTS

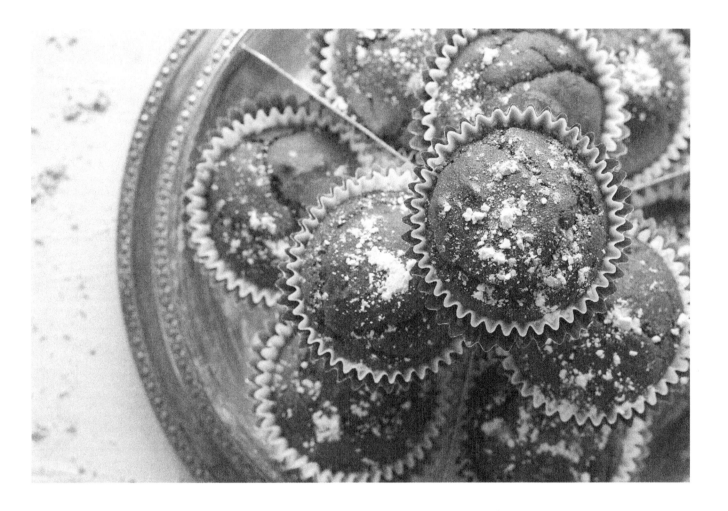

APPLE PIE FILLING

Preparation Time: 20 minutes
Cooking Time: 12 minutes
Servings: 40
Size/ Portion: 1 cup
Ingredients

- 18 cups chopped apples
- 3 tablespoons lemon juice
- 10 cups of water
- 4 1/2 cups of white sugar
- 1 cup corn flour
- 2 teaspoons of ground cinnamon
- 1 teaspoon of salt
- 1/4 teaspoon ground nutmeg

Direction

1. Mix apples with lemon juice in a large bowl and set aside. Pour the water in a Dutch oven over medium heat. Combine sugar, corn flour, cinnamon, salt, and nutmeg in a bowl. Add to water, mix well, and bring to a boil. Cook for 2 minutes with continuous stirring.
2. Boil apples again. Reduce the heat, cover, and simmer for 8 minutes. Allow cooling for 30 minutes.
3. Pour into five freezer containers and leave 1/2 inch of free space. Cool to room temperature.
4. Seal and freeze

Nutrition:
129 calories
0.1g fat
0.2g protein

ICE CREAM SANDWICH DESSERT

Preparation Time: 20 minutes
Cooking Time: 0 minute
Servings: 12
Size/ Portion: 2 squares
Ingredients

- 22 ice cream sandwiches
- Frozen whipped topping in 16 oz. container, thawed
- 1 jar (12 oz.) Caramel ice cream
- 1 1/2 cups of salted peanuts

Direction

1. Cut a sandwich with ice in two. Place a whole sandwich and a half sandwich on a short side of a 9 x 13-inch baking dish. Repeat this until the bottom is covered, alternate the full sandwich, and the half sandwich.
2. Spread half of the whipped topping. Pour the caramel over it. Sprinkle with half the peanuts. Do layers with the rest of the ice cream sandwiches, whipped cream, and peanuts.
3. Cover and freeze for up to 2 months. Remove from the freezer 20 minutes before serving. Cut into squares.

Nutrition:
559 calories 28.8g fat10g protein

CRANBERRY AND PISTACHIO BISCOTTI

Preparation Time: 15 minutes
Cooking Time: 35 minutes
Servings: 36
Size/ Portion: 2 slices
Ingredients

- 1/4 cup light olive oil

- 3/4 cup white sugar
- 2 teaspoons vanilla extract
- 1/2 teaspoon almond extract
- 2 eggs
- 1 3/4 cup all-purpose flour
- 1/4 teaspoon salt
- 1 teaspoon baking powder
- 1/2 cup dried cranberries
- 1 1/2 cup pistachio nuts

Direction

1. Prep oven to 150 ° C
2. Combine the oil and sugar in a large bowl until a homogeneous mixture is obtained. Stir in the vanilla and almond extract and add the eggs. Combine flour, salt, and baking powder; gradually add to the egg mixture — mix cranberries and nuts by hand.
3. Divide the dough in half — form two 12 x 2-inch logs on a parchment baking sheet. The dough can be sticky, wet hands with cold water to make it easier to handle it.
4. Bake in the preheated oven for 35 minutes or until the blocks are golden brown. Pullout from the oven and let cool for 10 minutes. Reduce oven heat to 275 degrees F (135 degrees C).
5. Cut diagonally into 3/4-inch-thick slices. Place on the sides on the baking sheet covered with parchment — Bake for about 8 to 10 minutes

Nutrition:
92 calories
4.3g fat
2.1g protein

CREAM PUFF DESSERT

Preparation Time: 20 minutes
Cooking Time: 36 minutes
Servings: 12
Size/ Portion: 2 puffs
Ingredients
Puff

- 1 cup water
- 1/2 cup butter
- 1 cup all-purpose flour
- 4 eggs

Filling

- 1 (8-oz) package cream cheese, softened
- 3 1/2 cups cold milk
- 2 (4-oz) packages instant chocolate pudding mix

Topping

- 1 (8-oz) package frozen whipped cream topping, thawed
- 1/4 cup topping with milk chocolate flavor
- 1/4 cup caramel filling
- 1/3 cup almond flakes

Direction:

1. Set oven to 200 degrees C (400 degrees F). Grease a 9 x 13-inch baking dish.
2. Melt the butter in the water in a medium-sized pan over medium heat. Pour the flour in one go and mix vigorously until the mixture forms a ball. Remove from heat and let stand for 5 minutes. Beat the eggs one by one until they are smooth and shiny. Spread in the prepared pan.
3. Bake in the preheated oven for 30 to 35 minutes, until puffed and browned. Cool completely on a rack.

4. While the puff pastry cools, mix the cream cheese mixture, the milk, and the pudding. Spread over the cooled puff pastry. Cool for 20 minutes.
5. Spread whipped cream on cooled topping and sprinkle with chocolate and caramel sauce. Sprinkle with almonds. Freeze 1 hour before serving.

Nutrition:
355 calories
22.3g fat
8.7g protein

CONCLUSION

There should be around 75% fat, 20% protein, and only 5% or less of 50 grams of carbs daily in a healthy ketogenic diet. Focus on fatty, low-carb foods such as eggs, meats, vegetables with milk and low carbon content as well as sugar-free drinks. Be sure that highly processed goods and unhealthy fats are prohibited.

Many of us are getting older, and, of course, death is imminent. Yet to a certain degree, we can monitor the quality of life along the way. People now live longer, but we get sicker by adopting the majority's normal diet. The ketogenic diet can help seniors improve their health so that they can thrive instead of being sick or suffering during their later lives.

This reduces the consumption of carbohydrate significantly and replaces it with fat. This decrease in carbon dioxide puts your body into metabolic state ketosis.

As this happens, the body uses fat for energy quite effectively. Fat also becomes ketones in the liver, which can supply the brain with energy.

Blood sugar and insulin levels can be reduced massively by ketogenic diets. In addition to the increased ketones, this has many health benefits.

The keto diet is a high-fat, low-carbon diet. It decreases blood sugar and insulin levels and eliminates the body metabolism from carbohydrates and to fat and ketones.

Printed in Great Britain
by Amazon

77008240R00093